D1507084

DR. SCOTT OLSON ND

SUGARETTES

Sugar Addiction and Your Health

DEDICATION

To my wife Tonya and my three children: Cody, Sasha and Sierra. Thank you for both abiding by, and supporting me, through the many hours I spent away from you writing and researching this book. And to My Parents, who always encouraged me to follow my dreams.

ACKNOWLEDGMENTS

I am grateful to all the eyes that have peeked over my shoulder and coaxed this book into a useful tool for the reader.

Thank you to my first editor Jo Urbanovitch, for her wise insights and her equally strong passions: good health and good grammar. To Judy Tomkins, for her medical expertise and her sharp eye that catches grammatical oddities that other eyes magically skip over. And to Sara Lynn Eastler of Atlantic Authoring for her amazing ability to create an index seemingly overnight, in addition to editing and improving the readability of the text. Thank you to Claire King and Brian Zimmerman for the work they have done on the layout of the book. And thank you to the whole crew at Booksurge who makes publishing a book seem easier than it really is.

Copyright © 2008 Wellbright LLC
All rights reserved.

ISBN: 1-4392-0276-1
ISBN-13: 9781439202760

Library of Congress Control Number: 2008906257

Visit www.booksurge.com to order additional copies.

Publishers note: The information contained in this book reflects the
author's personal experience and is not intended to take the place of, or
substitute for, medical or other health professionals advice. The intent
of this content is to offer information that will help you, along with the
aid of your health care provider, to make the best choices for you and
your health. Neither the authors, nor the publisher shall be held liable or
responsible for any loss or damage allegedly arising from any information
or suggestions contained within this book.

TABLE OF CONTENTS

INTRODUCTION

Addiction

When I tell people that I'm writing a book on the addictive properties of sugar, they nearly all admit that they too are addicted to the white stuff. When I tell them that I'm comparing eating sugar to smoking cigarettes, they all laugh. "Surely," they say, "I'm addicted to sugar, but there is no way that sugar is as harmful as cigarettes." Sugar, I have to tell them, is not as harmful, but actually much *more* harmful than cigarettes.

Have you ever wondered why so many foods contain sugar? Addiction is a powerful way to sell a product. Cigarette manufacturers have proven this is a strategy that works. But while cigarette companies have been held responsible for adding addictive substances to their cigarettes to ensure that you are a customer for life, food companies have been doing the same thing for decades and getting away with it. The next time you are in a grocery store, read the food labels on products you are buying, you will be astounded how many of the foods you have purchased contain sugar or high fructose corn syrup. Chances are your favorite foods are either sugar-laden foods or foods that act like sugar in your body.

Sugar has a real impact on your life whether you know it or not. If you have ever struggled to lose weight or have a disease such as diabetes or heart disease, sugar has had an impact on your life. If you find that you have extreme food cravings and have a tendency to binge on certain foods, sugar has had an impact on your life. If you have ever had an addiction, such as with cigarettes, alcohol, or other drugs, sugar has had an impact on your life. If you have felt weak and unable to change what you are eating, sugar has had an impact on your life.

When I began research for this book and discovered just how harmful sugar and foods that act like sugar can be, I decided to quit eating them, and, surprisingly, ran straight into my addiction. Most people who know me would say that I eat well and rarely eat table sugar, but the minute I stopped eating all sugar foods, something happened. I had intense cravings, felt ravenously hungry, would binge on all sorts of foods, and had bouts of grumpiness and a short temper. As you will learn throughout this book, these are the specific signs of an addiction and a withdrawal pattern seen so often with other equally addictive substances.

Sugar has a hold on us that is hard to break, but break it you must if you want to have a healthy and long life.

It has been suggested that we are on the verge of witnessing a generation of people who will have a shorter life span than their parents. Life expectancy, which slowly crept up from around forty years old in the 1900s to approximately seventy years old today, is beginning to slide backwards. Can this be possible? The next time you are at the store, the airport, a sporting event, or anywhere, take a look at the people around you. We just don't look so healthy.

The increase in obesity in the last few decades can only be called an epidemic. It doesn't seem like that long ago, but in 1990 less than ten percent of the people in the United States were considered obese. Today, that number is over thirty percent, with over sixty percent of the population who are not yet obese, but still considered overweight. If you ask people why they think they are overweight, they often shrug their shoulders and say, "I don't know. I am eating what the doctor tells me to eat." That, as you will find out, is the problem.

Where are we to lay the blame for this downward spiral in our health? Let's take a look.

Where Are You?

Imagine that you are in a waiting room at a doctor's office. A mother is standing, talking with a friend. Her young daughter, grabbing at her knee, is making it difficult for the two women to talk. The only words out of the little girl's mouth are "mommy, mommy, mommy." Her mother finally acknowledges her child, telling her that they will be leaving soon and that she has to wait. This sends the little girl into a rage. Her face turns red as tears pour down her face and she soon is screaming at the top of her lungs.

"Okay… okay," her mother finally says. She apologizes to her friend and reaches into her purse to grab a pack of cigarettes. The child immediately becomes quiet and is now focused on everything her mother is doing.

The mother lights the cigarette and holds it as the toddler takes a puff. The mother lets her take a few draws off the cigarette. After a few puffs, the mother tells her that she has had enough and she can have the rest later. Now content, the toddler lets go of her mother and turns to play with the blocks and toys on the floor.

Her mother returns to the conversation with her friend and saying, "She gets so fussy when I don't give her a smoke." Her friend nods knowingly and smiles, "Mine too, it is the only way I can force my kids to eat all their dinner. They know if they don't finish the green beans, they don't get their smoke."

The other mother nods knowingly.

Can't Happen Here

Imagine a whacky world where the above scene happens every day and no one notices. How strange it would be to live in that world. Imagine a Halloween where goblins and witches run door to door and shout "trick or treat" and people toss packages of cigarettes into their bags. Or what would Valentine's Day be like when your sweetheart sends you roses and a case of clove or menthol cigarettes, all in a pretty box?

Can't happen here? Right?

The reason it wouldn't happen here is because the dangers associated with smoking cigarettes are well known. This is true, but has it always been so?

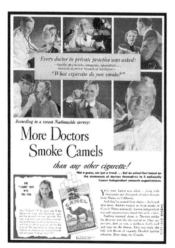

The answer is no; cigarettes were once considered not only not bad, but actually healthy. Incredible as it may seem today, family doctors and the prime-time 1960s cartoons, such as *The Flintstones,* used to promote cigarettes. It was only after decades of cigarette smoking and careful scientific research that the medical profession concluded cigarette smoking was something bad.

The reason doctors and *The Flintstones* thought cigarettes were healthy was because they made people feel good, alert, and calm: of course they were good for you.

But don't jump to blame the doctors too much; it was actually difficult to make the connection between smoking and lung cancer. There are good reasons why it was difficult to make this connection, but the most significant was the fact that smoking and the onset of lung cancer were separated by a large distance in time. It can take twenty or more years from that first puff to the dreaded diagnosis.

It took thousands of people "experimenting" with cigarettes until doctors and scientists came to the conclusion that cigarettes were bad for you. Hopefully, as a society, we've learned an important lesson. We do know enough not to give cigarettes to children in waiting rooms, on Halloween, or to our sweetheart, but we may not have learned all that we need to learn to be as healthy as we should be. Let's look at our other big addiction and see where it has taken us.

Shocking Sugar Stats

By tracking the amount of sugar people consume, it becomes clear that something dramatic has happened over the last one hundred years.

Sugar consumption at the beginning of the 1900s was very low; estimates suggest that people consumed about one pound of sugar per year. Astoundingly, today that number has risen to half a pound of sugar every **day**. This means that if you are typical, you eat more sugar in a week than your grandmother or great-grandmother did in an entire year.

When people hear this statistic, they simply can't imagine that they eat such an incredible amount of sugar. One half pound of sugar a day; are you sure? It's surprising, but true. If you consider all of the foods that contain sugar, you will see how easy it is to consume half a pound a day.

For example, ¼ pound of sugar is equal to around twenty-seven teaspoons. A typical twelve-ounce soda contains about ten teaspoons of sugar. If you drink two or three sodas each day, you have just consumed ¼ pound of sugar. And remember, those are small sodas (twelve ounce); many restaurants and gas station mini-marts serve much larger sodas. Now, add your soda sugar intake to any other candies, cookies, or other sweets that you eat. When you add in all the rest of the foods you eat that contain hidden sugar – including crackers, breads, ketchup, salad dressing, and so on – you can see how easy it is to meet your half a pound a day quota.

Sugar used to be expensive and hard to come by. It was like gold. In fact, during wartime, it was rationed. Now sugar is common and cheap. And because sugar is addictive, it is intentionally added to foods to keep you coming back for more.

Deadly Connection

It may come as a surprise, but sugar may cause as many deaths as cigarette smoking, perhaps even more. Let's start counting. If you consider that sugar is connected to diabetes (and not everyone does), the deaths caused by sugar and cigarettes are roughly the same. According to the World Health Organization, four million deaths a year are attributable to diabetes while smoking causes around five million deaths. But, as I will illustrate, sugar may be responsible for far more than four million diabetes deaths. Sugar may have links to obesity, heart disease, cancer, and other diseases. Factoring in all the deaths from these other sugar-related illnesses, the damage cigarettes cause is relatively small compared to sugar.

Yet, we ban cigarettes and allow soda and sugar-stocked vending machines in our schools.

Perhaps you are reacting the same way I did when I first began uncovering the truth about sugar. There was a disbelieving voice in the back of my head saying, "Oh, come on... eating sugar cannot possibly be as harmful as smoking cigarettes." Sugar is so safe that we *do* give it to little kids. It is in everything that we eat. It is natural, isn't it? How could it cause that much harm?

You are not alone in thinking this way. The medical community agrees with you; outside of dental problems, they don't think that sugar causes any harm at all. And that is what is really shocking; there is no one telling you the true harm that sugar can cause.

The doctors who first realized that there may be a connection between smoking and lung cancer were alone in their opinion. After all, everyone knew that smoking wasn't harmful. Were they crazy? Slowly, though, over time, the truth was revealed. Sugar sits at the same crossroads. Studies are beginning to show the link between sugar and obesity, diabetes, and heart disease. These studies are not enough to convince the medical community, but that will change. Despite sugar's overwhelming prevalence in our lives, human beings and sugar do not make very good bedfellows.

The Shoe-Toe Cancer Problem

You may wonder why no one in the medical community is sounding the alarm that sugar is harmful. The reasons are many and uncovering the link between sugar and the diseases it causes is much more difficult than finding the link between cigarettes and lung cancer.

There are two significant problems that make it difficult to pinpoint the harm done by sugar. The first is the same as the cigarette problem. It takes years for sugar-related health problems to make their presence known. If you drink a strong poison and end up in the emergency room, it is easy to connect the two. But if you are forty years old and forty pounds overweight and are sitting in front of your doctor with heart disease and diabetes, it is a tough task to pin this on the soda you have been drinking every day of your life.

The other difficulty has to do with finding a non-user's group. With cigarettes, it was relatively easy to find a group of people who didn't smoke. Naturally, some people smoke and others don't. All researchers had to do was compare smokers with non-smokers and wait. Decades later, it became a simple exercise to accurately predict who – between the two groups – was more likely to be diagnosed with lung cancer.

Finding a group of individuals who don't eat sugar is much more difficult. As we shall see, the challenge of finding a group of non-sugar-eaters is further complicated by the fact that many foods (like breads and other starches) act exactly like sugar in the blood stream. Finding people who don't eat any sugar or food that acts like sugar is a nearly impossible task in today's modern world.

To understand the enormity of this research problem, imagine what it would be like if wearing shoes caused toe cancer (this isn't true). How would we discover the truth? Most everyone in the world wears some type of foot covering, such as a sandal or a shoe. It would be very difficult to find a non-shoe-wearing population that we could compare to our shoe-wearing society.

If there was an epidemic of people with toe cancer, scientists may start by thinking that the cancer could be caused by shoes but not sandals or by high-heeled shoes, but not tennis shoes. It would be a big step to think that toe cancer may be caused by something almost everyone does: wearing shoes. Scientists suffer from the same blindness we all have; it is hard to question something that everyone is doing.

This is the exact problem we face when trying to determine whether or not sugar foods cause health problems. Most people in the world eat sugar or foods that act like sugar, or both. This makes finding a non-user's group very difficult.

Our medical professionals are not sounding the alarm about sugar; they have yet to compare the sugary foods that we eat with the foods that humans should be eating. They typically compare sugar to sugar foods (bread and other starches) and see no difference in how these foods affect our blood sugar, our diseases, and our health. No wonder! They are comparing shoe-wearing to sandal-wearing and not seeing any difference in the rates of toe cancer. What they really need to find is a group of bare-footed people and see how many of them have toe cancer. This book is about finding those bare-footed people, those who don't eat sugar or foods that act like sugar. To do this, though, we have some traveling to do.

Let's start our journey to uncover the truth about sugar by taking a short detour to uncover how our attitudes toward cigarettes have changed over time.

The History of Cigarettes

Cigarettes, of course, are made from tobacco. As far as scientists can determine, tobacco is native to the Americas and was smoked long before the Europeans arrived. It wasn't long after tobacco was "discovered" that it spread throughout the entire world. At first, people smoked whole leaf tobacco in a pipe; eventually it was packaged and sold in cigarette form for convenience.

Remember, cigarettes were originally thought to be healthy. Think about that; not neutral like drinking water, but actually good for our health. We thought that cigarettes were healthy because they produce mental and physical changes. People feel more alert, calmer, and get a boost of energy when they smoke.

Hmm…sound familiar? Doesn't sugar give you energy?

The good feelings that smoking cigarettes create belies the hidden destruction occurring in smokers' lungs. Cigarette companies donated cigarettes to World War I soldiers for free. Cigarettes were also included in World War II rations. Many soldiers returned from war addicted to cigarettes and were the first large population to embrace the habit.

Around 1930 (20 years after World War I), doctors began to notice a dramatic rise in people with lung cancer and pondered what was causing the increase.

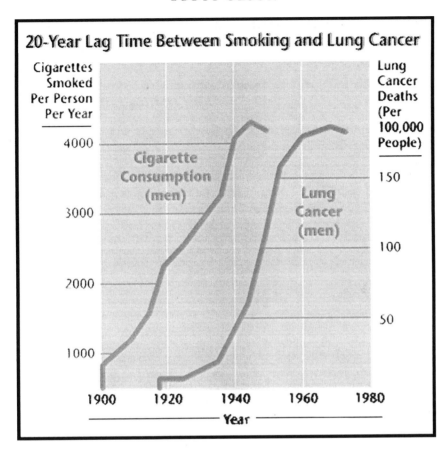

The older doctors could remember a time when lung cancer was rare; in fact, it was an almost non-existent disease before 1900. An extremely rare disease was now becoming commonplace. Something had changed, but what?

Studies started to suggest that cigarettes may be the cause of the rising lung cancer rates, but it was not until twenty years later, in 1950, that the definitive studies blaming the rise in lung cancer on cigarettes began to appear.

Now we look back and feel silly; of course, cigarettes cause lung cancer. Today we can blame lung cancer, emphysema, heart disease, stroke, and other diseases squarely on cigarette smoking.

Still, the connection between diseases and smoking was difficult to make. What cigarettes had going for them was that lung cancer was rare. Once enough time had passed, it was easy to connect lung cancer to cigarette smoking. But think about this; even though it was a rare disease *and* there was a clear non-user's group, it still took almost fifty years to connect smoking to disease.

As we shall see, the number of people who are overweight has grown dramatically in the past decades, along with the number of people with diabetes and heart disease, but no one is blaming anything for these increases; at least not yet.

No Disease Connection

This is the point in the book where I show you that there is absolutely no connection between sugar and any disease (well, except for dental cavities, and that can be solved by brushing). That is, there is no connection if you believe the current medical wisdom.

Understand what I am saying: There is no major medical association, scientific body, or governmental group that states there is anything wrong with sugar in our diet. A few health agencies may issue warnings about the *amount* of sugar in our diet, but no one is saying that you should stop eating sugar. None of these groups are connecting sugar to any disease.

Obviously, the sugar industry couldn't be happier with what the medical community has to say about sugar. To get an idea of how strong the evidence is against the connection between diseases and sugar, let's take a peek at the sugar industry's website (www.sugar.org):

Starting with its 1986 review of 1000 scientific papers, the Food and Drug Administration's (FDA) Sugars Task Force in their report on "Evaluation of Health Aspects of Sugars contained in Carbohydrate Sweeteners" reported that "with the exception of dental caries [cavities], the scientific evidence clears sugars of links with other diseases including diabetes, hypertension, behavior and obesity." [1]

This seems like pretty definitive evidence: Over 1000 scientific papers and a special task force in the Food and Drug Administration concluded that there is no link between sugar and diabetes, hypertension, behavior, or obesity. Sounds like it is okay to eat sugar, don't you think? The sugar industry is also happy to report that there is no such thing as a sugar "high" or a sugar "crash" despite how you feel after you eat a lot of sugar. They also report that children do not experience mood shifts or become hyperactive when they eat sugar, even though any parent would tell you differently.

The sugar industry also has a lot to say about the connection between sugar and diabetes. Here, on their website, they quote from the American Diabetes Association:

Does Sugar Cause Diabetes?

There is no reason to be concerned that if your child eats sugar it will lead to diabetes.

Normally, carbohydrates in the foods we eat are digested and changed into glucose, the sugar that circulates in the blood and is one of the body's major sources of energy. Before the body can use glucose as energy, insulin (a hormone produced by the pancreas) must be present to allow body tissue to convert glucose to energy.

A person with diabetes either does not produce enough insulin or cannot properly use the insulin the pancreas does produce. According to the American Diabetes Association, sugar does not cause diabetes.

Not only does sugar not cause diabetes but individuals with diabetes do not have to strictly avoid eating sugar according to the American Diabetes Association:

"The available evidence from clinical studies demonstrates that dietary sucrose does not increase glycemia more than isocaloric amounts of starch. Thus, intake of sucrose and sucrose containing foods by people with diabetes does not need to be restricted because of concern about aggravating hyperglycemia. Sucrose should be substituted for other carbohydrate sources in the food/meal plan or, if added to the food/meal plan, adequately covered with insulin or other glucose-lowering medication."[2]

In truth, there is no blaming the sugar industry or the American Diabetes Association. After all, it is scientific study that guides their decisions and there is currently not enough scientific research to change their minds. The reason there is not enough research to change minds of the American Diabetes Association is that scientists doing the research are still not asking the right questions (remember the toe cancer problem?). Scientists, for the most part, are comparing sugar to other carbohydrates and seeing no difference in what happens to our blood sugar or the amount of disease these foods cause.

The research connecting sugar foods to diseases is growing and may soon be enough to change even the minds of the medical community. But let's take a closer look at the above quote from the sugar industry website to see exactly what they are saying. They say, *"The available evidence from clinical studies demonstrates that dietary sucrose does not increase glycemia more than isocaloric amounts of starch."* In layman's terms, this means that table sugar does not increase glycemia (blood sugar) more than isocaloric amounts of starch (identical amounts of calories from other starches). What this means is that sugar does not raise your blood sugar more than eating, say, white bread.

This is absolutely true, but what the sugar industry and American Diabetes Association don't admit is that there are two conclusions to be drawn from noticing that white bread and sugar act identically in the body.

The first is the conclusion that they made: Since table sugar and other starches act the same in the body, there is no need to avoid sugar. The question that the sugar industry and medical community are not asking, however, is this: Should these foods be in our bodies at all? Is there a problem with both sugar and sugar foods that can lead to disease in humans?

As we shall see, comparing table sugar to these isocaloric starches is exactly like asking if there is any difference between tennis shoes and sandals for our people with toe cancer. Of course there is no difference between the two – sugars and many starches act identically in your body. I will explain exactly what "isocaloric starches" are later and discuss the important role they play in obesity, diabetes, and your general health.

It is good to remember that when people first started using cigarettes, no one questioned the alleged health benefits of smoking, even though it now seems absurd to think that tobacco could provide health benefits. It was decades before the connection between cigarettes and lung cancer was made. There was, however, an explosion of research once that connection was made.

Today, the dangers of smoking are common knowledge. This is where I think we are headed with sugar. We are just beginning to question the relationship between what goes into our mouths and the current pandemic of chronic diseases.

Sugar is harmful and it is addictive. While the research to support this fact is just beginning to surface, it continues to grow in strength. As with any new area of study, the evidence from current study outcomes may not always be convincing on its own. But when you string together the pieces from many different studies, an obvious pattern is beginning to emerge and take shape. You and sugar foods need to part ways.

Diabetes Leads the Way

I'll use the rise in the number of people with diabetes throughout this book as a marker for evidence of the harmful effects of sugar on human beings, just as we now use the statistics on lung cancer as a marker for the harmful effects of smoking. While this is sure to be controversial, there is good reason to think that sugar and foods that act like sugar can lead to diabetes.

I wish I could show you a chart created by a reputable organization showing the relationship between sugar consumption and the rate of diabetes. No one has created this chart yet because the connection is not believed to be real. There is, however, a National Health Interview Surveys graph that clearly illustrates the dramatic rise in the number of people with diabetes over the last fifty years.

The graph illustrates that diabetes has been steadily increasing for five decades, from less than one percent of the population

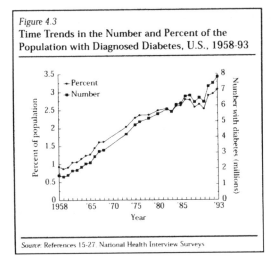

Figure 4.3
Time Trends in the Number and Percent of the
Population with Diagnosed Diabetes, U.S., 1958-93

Source: References 15-27. National Health Interview Surveys

to nearly four percent of the population.

Hmm...diabetes has been increasing for the last fifty years. Remember, the rate of sugar consumption was very low around 1900 and then began to rise until we now have people today eating around 150 pounds of sugar a year. Is it merely a coincidence that both diabetes and sugar consumption have skyrocketed in the last fifty years?

Powerful Combination

The problem with sugar and cigarettes is that they are both highly addictive as well as harmful. This is a powerful, and potentially devastating, combination for anything you want to put into your body.

Remember the first scene of this book? Do you remember the mother and her child in the doctor's office? Try replacing the cigarettes in that setting with some sugar food, like a lollipop or a soda. That scene is so common that you have probably witnessed something like it every day and don't even notice. We use sugar as a reward and a celebration, not only for our children but for ourselves. Sugar is our most common mood-altering substance. How often have you felt down, tired, or cranky and reached for a soda or a chocolate bar? It is clear that we use sugar in ways that we don't use other foods. Can you imagine reaching for broccoli to make you feel better when you are sad?

While proving that sugar is an addiction can be a difficult task, try taking this little addiction quiz to see how addicted you are to sugars:

- Have you ever used sugar as a reward for something?
- Have you ever used sugar to change your mood, like when you felt sad, tired, or when you needed a lift?
- Have you ever eaten sugar even when you weren't hungry?
- Have you ever tried to stop eating sugar and couldn't?
- Have you ever taken a small bite of something sweet and felt compelled to finish the whole thing?
- Have you ever banished sugar and carbohydrates from your diet, but began eating them again because you couldn't resist the pull they had on you?
- Have you ever quit eating sugar and when you started eating it again, couldn't stop binging?

If you answered no to all of the above questions, you can put this book down and walk away. If not, read on. I have a lot to tell you about your relationship with sugar and what to do to make that relationship not so harmful. This book is about understanding how and why sugar has a strange grip on us. It is about how you can reduce or eliminate sugar from your life or, at the very least – if you can't kick the sugar habit – how you can reduce the impact it may have on your health.

Thinking the Next Thought

Imagine how surprised you would be if you walked into a pet store, as I did a few years ago, and found a nutritional genius! My family and I were choosing our first dog and the clerk who was helping us mentioned that the breed of dog we had chosen was especially susceptible to diabetes. She looked at us in a scolding manner and said, "You do know how to keep this dog from getting diabetes, don't you?" She paused, waiting for us to answer.

Even though I had studied health and nutrition all my life and had recently graduated from naturopathic school,[1] I was, for once, speechless on the subject of health. I shrugged my shoulders and waited in anticipation. What secret knowledge did she have; some miracle cure?

After waiting for us to answer, she finally said, "Keep your dog away from people food and she will never get diabetes."

This cashier at the pet store, with no formal training in nutrition, appeared to know more about human nutrition than most medical doctors, scientists, and nutritionists (including me). While the girl in the pet store knew definitively that human food caused diabetes in dogs, she didn't take the time to think the next thought: *that she isn't all that different from a dog.* She was young, but she was very overweight, and had an extra-large soda and French fries sitting on the counter next to the cash register.

Thinking the next thought is hard, but it is also an essential tool for your health. For example, you may know that sugar is bad for your teeth, but, somehow, it is still okay to eat. How

---

1   For more about what a naturopathic doctor is, see the end of the book

can this be? Shouldn't we get the hint that sugar isn't the best food to put in our bodies if it is responsible for destroying our teeth (one of the hardest substances in the human body)? If we were meant to eat sugars, shouldn't our teeth be able to handle them?

The scientific community, of course, does admit that sugar causes cavities. Scientists are now grudgingly starting to think that there may be a connection between the sugar we eat and obesity. But thinking that sugar is actually the cause of diseases, such as diabetes, heart disease, or cancer is much too great a leap for them to make.

The large rise in blood sugar that occurs when we eat sugar and foods that act like sugar is not natural for human beings. To understand why this is so, we would have to go back in time. Think about what would happen if you were suddenly dropped into a time machine and ended up in a field 10,000 years ago. No farms, no large cities; just you, your bare hands, and the world around you. What would you eat? No processed foods, no concentrated sugars (unless you want to fight the bees for their honey), no preservatives, and no packaged anything.

While your mind may be confused by this trip into the past, your body would rejoice. This is the world that your body understands: whole foods, clean air, and fresh water. I am in no way advocating that we all go back to the caveman's world – there are too many advantages to the world we live in – but we need to appreciate and understand what our bodies need as we attempt to navigate our contemporary world.

Research

S. Boyd Eaton, MD, a researcher who has studied how human diets have changed over time, describes the dilemma we all face:

> *As a rule, organisms are healthiest when their life circumstances most closely approximate the conditions for which their genes were selected.*[3]

Seems simple enough, but the problem is that we live far from the life circumstances for which our genes were selected. Most of the foods that we put into our mouths are very different from the way that they are found in nature. This is no small point. What you put into your mouth does matter. Instead of giving our bodies the foods we need, we eat what is convenient, fast, and tasty. Eating this way is a recipe for obesity and disease. While the foods that we eat have indeed changed since we dwelled in caves, the most dramatic change in our diets has happened fairly recently, during the last 100 years or so. The foods we eat have changed from locally produced home-cooked meals to a marketed product that is designed for taste and shelf life.

Some researchers have started looking for those "shoeless" people in our "toe cancer" example and believe they have found them. There are still people on this planet who live what we would call a traditional hunter-gatherer existence. Upon examination, these traditional peoples are free of many of the diseases that we find so common in our modern world. High blood pressure, obesity, high cholesterol, and blood sugar problems are almost non-existent in hunter-gatherer societies.[4] We have a lot to learn for traditional cultures.

There is a new type of dietary thinking developing that suggests that our bodies have evolved over millions of years along *with* and *next to* the foods we eat. The minute we planted grains, though, we changed the game. As you will see, agriculture equals processed foods; after all, how long would you survive eating the grains we grow straight from the field? Whether we are simply grinding the grains to make bread or using them to create Chocolate Yoo-Hoos, grains must somehow be processed in order for us to eat them.

As we will discover, eating processed grains and sugars ensures that your blood sugar will rise to a level that can be harmful to your body.

The overall problem is that we have modified and processed our foods faster than our genes have been able to adapt. We still have the bodies of our cave-dwelling ancestors, but we are eating foods that are far from the foods they ate. The result is that we live in a world surrounded by diseases that we assume are a normal part of human life, when the reality is, many of these diseases are a result of what we choose to put on our dinner plates.

You now know from my friend at the pet shop to keep human food away from your dog if you want to keep your pet healthy, but what are you going to do about the food you choose to put into your own mouth?

The Road Ahead

This book will trace the history of sugar and how it evolved from a luxury to a common food additive. We will see what happens when sugar enters our bloodstream and how our body reacts to it. We will also look at the addictive properties of sugars and foods that act like sugar, as well as the diseases these sugar foods may cause. Sugar addiction not only explains why we consume as much sugar as we do, but also why we have a hard time giving up sugar and even why we have a difficult time losing weight.

This book is not strictly a health book. I'm not going to give you recipes or a meal plan. I will, however, give you suggestions about how you can eliminate sugar and foods that act like sugar in your body from your diet. If this is too great a step for you, I can also show you ways to minimize the damage of sugar without giving it up completely.

Your body is wondrous. When you give your body what it needs, it responds with good health. If you implement the suggestions outlined in this book, you will feel better, sleep more deeply, have more energy, and even look better. And, yes, if you want to lose weight, adapting my program will help you with that too.

The reason sugar is much more harmful than cigarettes is that no one is sounding the alarm. People know that cigarettes are bad, so they can choose to avoid them. Public education about the harm that cigarettes cause is what has accounted for the dramatic drop in lung cancer rates, especially in Western countries. My hope is that sugar takes its place alongside cigarettes and is considered to be a major risk to your good health. Sugar is a powerfully concentrated food that ought to be understood as potentially harmful and should be consumed with caution, rather than something to be had with every meal.

Today, as in no other time in the history of humanity, we have the means to provide our body with exactly what it needs to truly thrive. Don't miss this opportunity to make the most out of your life.

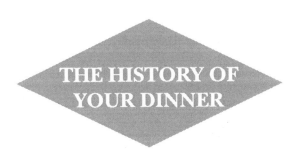

THE HISTORY OF YOUR DINNER

Okay, let's take you out of the strange whacky world where children smoke and sweethearts exchange fancy cigarettes for Valentine's Day. Let's instead, take a trip to an even stranger place... your local restaurant.

Imagine that tonight you are out to dinner with friends and family. You have chosen a local restaurant and, unbeknownst to you and your party, you are about to take the ride of a lifetime. The waitress walks up to your table with a smile and asks what you would like to order. You scan the menu and choose something. After everyone at the table has ordered, your waitress thanks you and tells you that your meals will be here shortly. You and your dinner companions return to talking about the day's events.

After awhile your smiling waitress returns with your order. She sets the hot meals all around the table. The food looks and smells great. But, despite what your eyes and nose are telling you, there is something wrong. Can you figure it out? To you and your dinner companions, nothing looks out of place; in fact, it all looks perfectly normal. But let's take a closer look and see if we can find out what is amiss.

On the table are a variety of meals. Someone ordered a hamburger and fries, another person ordered spaghetti and meatballs, and someone else had the chicken with vegetables, and so on. Drinks include a chocolate shake, sodas, and maybe a beer or glass of wine.

Nothing wrong here, huh?

The foods in front of you are exactly the kind of meals you grew up with; everyone you know eats pretty much the same kinds of foods you see on the table. As far as you know, this is exactly what your parents ate, and their parents ate, and their parents, and so on... There is a tendency to think that the way that you (and human beings in general) are eating today is the way human beings have always eaten. After all, pasta, hamburgers, chicken, soda, beer, and wine have been around forever, haven't they?

Well, yes and no. Let's take pasta, for example.

Pasta has a long history, but not as long as you may think. While there is a legend about Marco Polo bringing pasta to Europe, this isn't true. The Italians have been making pasta for around 2,000 years (well before Marco Polo's journey). The earliest known mention of pasta anywhere in the world is around 4,000 years ago in a Chinese text. That means that pasta has been around for at least a few thousand years, but its use was limited and the bulk of the world didn't start eating it until much later. Thomas Jefferson is credited with bringing the first macaroni machine to America in 1789, but pasta wasn't manufactured on a large scale until the 1850s. So in real terms, pasta that was easily available to everyone has only been around 150 years or so. While this may seem like a long time – and surely 4,000 years of pasta history seems significant – in terms of human history and, more importantly, in terms of your biology, 4,000 years is barely a blip on the cosmic calendar.

So, getting back to your dinner with friends, what is wrong with the food at your table? You recognize it as food, but your body may have a hard time understanding and digesting these relatively new processed foods. To fully understand the significance of this, we need to go on a journey. So grab a bite of your dinner because you are about to take a trip, not to a someplace but to a *somewhen.*

A man with a strange hat and a small hand-held device walks up to your table with an offer you cannot refuse. "How would you like to take a trip back in time?" he asks. You look around the table at your dinner companions and shrug your shoulders. Half-joking, you say, "Sure, why not?" The man asks for $10 from each of you, and you willingly pay the token fee... an incredible bargain for time travel, you think. The man with the hat grabs a chair and sits down at your table and sets his machine on your table. To you, the machine looks like a cell phone, nothing fancy. He adjusts his hat, pokes at some of the buttons, and the machine begins to make a funny sound. At first nothing happens, but soon you notice the people in the room freeze and begin to move backwards. The clock on the wall stops and begins a counterclockwise spin. You grab on to the table, not really believing what is happening.

A Little Grocery Store in Time

The man with the machine calls your attention back to the table. He leans over to tell you that while you and your dinner table will move back in time; objects will continue to exist in front of you only as long as they can be found in the current time. "For example," he explains, "your cell phone will disappear around 1973 when they were first invented." And sure enough, as you watch the date on the time machine spin back from today to 1990, then 1980, your cell phone starts to fade and eventually disappears as you approach 1970. "Don't worry," he explains with a smile, "You will get your phone back when we return to your normal time." A little relieved, you sit back and relax, but then you notice something odd; as you approach 1930, the food on the table is starting to fade.

The first things to go are the drinks. Coca-Cola, Pepsi, and Dr. Pepper and other sodas were all invented around 1880, but it took a while until bottling made them widely available outside the soda fountain. By 1920, most people could easily find a soda whenever they were thirsty. As the journey backwards in time continues, other foods begin to fade. Your hamburger leaves the table around 1890; french fries and the pasta vanish around 1850. When the machine reaches 1800, not one of your meals is left at the table. Remember, this is only two hundred years ago and all that is left are the salad greens, vegetables, meat, water, beer, and wine.

Now that we are in 1800 and your plate is empty, the man in the funny hat smiles and says for an extra twenty dollars each he could let you take a walk outside the restaurant and experience what 1800 looks like. You laugh as you now understand how this guy makes his money, but you are curious, so you agree. You step up from your table and leave the restaurant, walking onto a bustling street. The first thing you notice is the lack of lights and advertisements that fill our modern cities. As you peek in shop windows, you notice that there is no refrigeration, no televisions, no phones, or radios. While you hear the hooves of horses on the street, there is little other noise.

You walk across a street and enter a general store.

What you will find as you walk into the store is that there are plenty of foods that you recognize, but not a lot of it is packaged. A funny thought occurs to you; while you recognize everything you see in this small store, someone from this time would be baffled by your grocery store. Sure, they would recognize everything on the edges of a modern grocery store: the dairy section, the meat and produce section, but everything in the center of the store – cereals, frozen foods, chips, boxes, bags and containers of food – would all be unrecognizable, since most food from the 1800s was homemade.

Let's take another little detour and look at some of the foods we consider common and see how long they have been around. While the origin of many foods is hotly debated, these are the general dates when these foods were introduced into our diets.

1924: Frozen foods first appeared
1890: Pizza
1870: Hot dogs
1860: Breakfast cereals
1850: Potato chips
1850: Donuts
1850: French Fries

Standing back in the store here in 1800, what can you eat? Put another way, what can you find to eat that *you normally eat?* Where are your breakfast cereals, bread, ice cream, soda, yogurt, sandwich or the chocolate chip cookies you like to snack on? Do you find it a little strange that nothing you are used to eating is here and yet you have only traveled back 200 years? Here in 1800, the major preservatives are salt, vinegar, and drying. Food coloring, additives, and preservatives aren't introduced for another century. Your taste buds would be bored with many of the food choices here in the 1800s because food manufacturers have yet to learn what really sends your taste buds reeling... the addictive little additives that keep you coming back for more.

But here is what is really going to surprise you; your body is still confused. Even though we have traveled back over 200 years and removed many of the modern additives and processing from our foods, we still haven't found the foods that match our genes. Let's end our tour of the grocery store and return to our dinner table and see where the time machine will take us next.

Going Way Back

Back at your dinner table, the man with the time machine punches his buttons and adjusts dials. The time machine comes to life again and further back in time you go. As you approach the year 1500, something remarkable happens. On the table, the tomatoes in the salad fade and disappear. The 1500s must have been an incredible time to be alive. Columbus set sail in 1492 and that voyage set off an explosion of exploration to the so-called New World. With the increase in exploration came a vast array of foods that most of the world had never seen before. Imagine what the world would have been like without potatoes, corn, tomatoes, beans, pumpkins, strawberries, or peanuts. All of these, and more, came from the New World.

As the time machine sends you even further in time, wine and beer begin to fade about 7,000 years ago. Beer is the oldest known processed food on the planet and is the last to fade from the table.

A few more millennia and you and your table companions arrive in a field, 10,000 years ago. You are struck by the silence as you look around at the empty open field. Ten thousand years ago is a long way to travel in time. There were no large cities anywhere on earth and no one is farming foods at this point in history. If you thought it was difficult to find something to eat back in 1800, try to find something to eat now! What are you going to put into your mouth when you are hungry?

That is a good question: What are we going to eat?

While your mind is likely baffled by your trip into the very distant past, your body has finally arrived where it feels comfortable. Fresh air, clean water, foods that don't contain preservatives – none of the food that you find here would confuse your body. Here, 10,000 years ago, our genetic makeup matches our environment.

Anthropologists agree that human beings were at one time hunter-gatherers. Then, somewhere around 10,000 years ago, we started to grow grains. This field where the time machine has stopped is a critical junction for human beings. From here, on into the present, we made two critical choices. First, we began eating grains and sugars in increasingly larger amounts and we began changing and processing our foods. No longer did we simply eat foods the way that they were presented to us in nature. We began grinding grains and making breads and alcoholic drinks. From there, we moved to our modern grocery store and restaurants where we eat very few foods the way they are naturally found.

Think about what a profound change we made to our diets. The so-called agricultural revolution began 10,000 years ago, but didn't really get going until about 7,000 years ago. Before that, we only ate food that we could dig up or catch. Ten thousand years may seem like a long time to adapt to a new diet, but it is simply not enough time for your genes to adapt to a new way of eating. As we shall see, this move from hunting and gathering to grain and sugar eating may not have been the best choice for us.

Not the Right Foods

How do we know that the switch to agriculture may not have been the best choice for us? Anthropologists who dig up the remains of our ancestors, and those who follow modern human beings who have made the switch from a hunter-gatherer existence to agriculturally-based diets, have noticed something startling. When people change from a low-carbohydrate diet to a high-carbohydrate diet, they are much less healthy than their ancestors who ate a traditional diet. The people who switch their diets typically lose height (up to six to eight inches), have shorter life spans, more tooth decay, osteoporosis, and even have an increased incidence of infectious diseases than their ancestors.

Imagine if you were a gardener and you tried an experiment in which you planted two identical plants in two different pots. In one of the pots you tried a new nutritional formula, and in the other you used traditional plant food. If after a few months you noticed that the plant given the traditional food grew very large and the other one was stunted and full of disease, wouldn't you conclude that the traditional diet was optimal and the new one wasn't?

This is exactly the conclusion of a growing number of scientists who believe that our genes are adapted to the foods found in the fields of 10,000 years ago and, as a result, our bodies are simply unable to handle much of what we put in our mouths today.

This type of thinking is called Evolutionary Health Promotion.[1] Here are two main points of this thinking:

- The human genome was selected in past environments far differently from those of the present.
- Cultural evolution now proceeds too rapidly for genetic accommodation, resulting in dissociation between our genes and our lives.

In other words, our genes and our bodies are simply not being fed what they need in order to function optimally and that much of the disease we see in modern life has to do with the foods we eat. The most problematic of these foods are the sugars and foods that act like sugar that we put into our bodies every day.

Nutritional Tipping Points

While there are plenty of reasons not to stay in a field some 10,000 years ago, this is the exact place you need to think about when you find yourself faced with the question of what to put on your plate. We have come a long way in the last 10,000 years, our world is full of opportunities and advances that ought to spell better health for all of us; instead, the opposite is true. While we have seen progress in many areas of human health and medicine, our nutritional choices have only gotten worse over time.

What could you eat if you were stuck here 10,000 years ago? All you have are your bare hands and no tools? Answering that question is one of the key steps toward good health and longevity. I will have suggestions about how to make this work for you later in the book.

During your trip back through time, you witnessed four pivotal "tipping points" in human nutrition. The first one occurred when we dropped our spears and picked up a plow. The second one was around 1500 when the world began getting smaller as explorers spread out over the globe and discovered new foods to share with the world. Many of these – corn, tomatoes, and potatoes, for example – make up a large proportion of our diets.

The third major change to our diet occurred about 200 years ago when store-bought food began to take the place of homemade food; this marked the start of the industrial manufacturing of our food.

The fourth and final change occurred sometime after World War II. These were perhaps the most damaging changes – sugar, preservatives, colorings, and the institutionalization of the food –were implemented. Prepared meals, frozen dinners, and fast food restaurants, that were once a rarity, became commonplace.

Notice that as time has passed, more and more people (and machines) have come between you and your food. In the past, we picked up a piece of food and ate it. Today there are multiple steps that food must undergo before it makes it to your mouth: from people picking and harvesting, to processing and preparing, to transporting. Food takes an incredibly long and transformative journey before it ever arrives on your plate.

You should remember this: The greater the number of people and/or machines touching your food before you, the farther away food is from being whole and natural.

Eating the way that we eat has created a scientific experiment of sorts. We now are putting more carbohydrates in our bodies in a day than our pre-historic ancestors would probably encounter in their entire lifetimes. The results of this experiment are the chronic diseases you see every day. Eating sugar and foods that act like sugar has real consequences for your body and we will look into those consequences as we move through the rest of the book.

Back Home

One last time, the man with the time machine punches his buttons and adjusts his dials and you end up back where you started...cell phone, dinner, and all. He stuffs the money you paid him into his shirt pocket, tips his hat, gets up from the table, and walks away.

After your journey through time, you may be left wondering if you should finish your meal, but go ahead. We have a bit further to go before we begin suggesting what you may want to eat and what you may want to avoid. The next journey you are going to take is a place you thought you would never end up again.

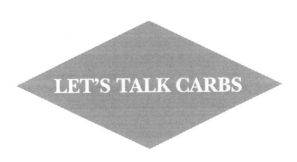

LET'S TALK CARBS

This book has been a journey. You have already been on a ride to a strange, cigarette-laden land and a trip back through time. While those journeys may have been somewhat enjoyable, the place I am going to take you now is somewhere you probably thought you would never go again.

On this next trip, I'm going to take you back to your high school science class. I'm going to bring you back to high school because I'm guessing that you were sleeping when your teacher gave the carbohydrate talk. Of all the classes you could have slept through, the carbohydrate class was not your best choice! You probably hear about carbohydrates daily and may even use the word in conversation. But even though carbohydrate is a common word, most people don't really understand what exactly a carbohydrate is or what it does in your body. Knowing what carbohydrates are is crucial to our sugar tale; sugar is, after all, the king of carbohydrates.

In this high school science class, we will look at the chemical structure of carbohydrates, understand what they are, and discover the difference between simple and complex carbohydrates.

You may be tempted to skip this class and move on with the rest of the book, and I really couldn't blame you if you did! But why don't you resist that temptation and see if you can squeeze back into that uncomfortable school chair, stop day-dreaming or writing notes, and pay attention to the teacher this time? Understanding carbohydrates will help you to also understand how they act in your body.

I'll try and make it as painless as possible.

What is a Carbohydrate?

Strictly speaking, a carbohydrate is a carbon atom (C), a hydrogen atom (H), and an oxygen atom (O), arranged in various configurations. Carbohydrates get much more complex than this, but carbon, hydrogen, and oxygen is all it takes to build a basic carbohydrate. If you attach a carbon atom to a hydrate (H_2O or water) molecule, you get a carbohydrate. The name comes from combining the words *carbon* and *hydrate:* carbon hydrate, carbo-hydrate, or – as you know it – sugar, rice, bread, or pasta. Today, the foods we consider to be carbohydrates are not all strictly carbon-hydrates, but the name stuck and this is what we use.

Combining carbon, hydrogen, and oxygen atoms together creates every carbohydrate we know. For example, six carbon atoms, twelve hydrogen atoms, and six oxygen atoms combine to make one of the simplest sugars: glucose. In scientific notation, glucose looks like this: $C_6H_{12}O_6$. That white stuff that you pour on your morning cereal, otherwise known as sucrose or table sugar, looks like this: $C_{12}H_{22}O_{11}$.

All carbohydrates come from one place: the sun. A carbohydrate is produced in plants and some animals by a process called photosynthesis. This process takes the energy from sunlight and transforms it into food energy. All life on earth stems from this conversion of sunlight into energy.

So, you still with me, class?

Carbohydrates come in many different sizes or lengths. The simplest versions of carbohydrates are known as monosaccharides. You can break down the word "monosaccharide" to understand what it means. Mono means "single" or "one" and saccharide means "sugar." You are probably familiar with some monosaccharides, such as glucose and fructose. Other less commonly known monosaccharides are galactose, xylose, ribose, and others. Chemically, monosaccharides take on a specific shape, but since they are considered the building blocks of all other carbohydrates, it helps to imagine them as blocks.

So, glucose and fructose molecules could look like this:

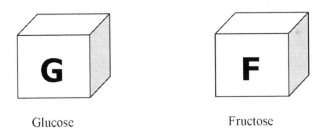

Glucose   Fructose

Now that we have the basic carbohydrate building blocks, let's see what we can do with them.

The next carbohydrates up the ladder of complexity are called disaccharides (di meaning "two" and saccharide meaning "sugar"). These carbohydrates are molecules that have two sugars linked to each other. You may also be familiar with many of these: lactose, sucrose, maltose, and others. To build a disaccharide, you simply combine the basic building blocks (monosaccharides) together. Table sugar (or sucrose) is the combination of glucose and fructose molecules and maltose is the combination of two glucose molecules. Using our blocks, they would look like this:

Sucrose   Maltose

From here on out, all we have to do is string a bunch of sugar molecules together to get all the rest of the carbohydrates.

If we stitch together between three and twenty different sugars or saccharides, we get what are called the oligosaccharides. Examples of oligosaccharides are inulin and fructooligosaccharides (FOS). These are unique carbohydrates because we only partially digest most of them and they end up being digested by the bacteria in our gut.

An oligosaccharide might look something like this:

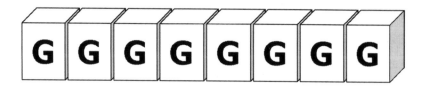

Polysaccharides (poly meaning "many" and saccharide meaning "sugar"), with more than twenty sugar building blocks per string, make up the rest of the carbohydrates. These carbohydrates are much more chemically complex and can have many branched chains – like a tree's branches – making it difficult for our body's digestive forces to tear them apart. Being difficult to digest doesn't mean that these carbohydrates don't play a role in the body. We know many of these hard-to-digest carbohydrates as fiber, cellulose, and gums which add bulk to our stools.

Okay, did you get all of that, or are you are sleeping in the back of the class again? Why don't you wake up for just a few more moments, grab your pencil, and jot these important points down for the upcoming test? We had to go through all that basic science in order to understand some fundamental points about carbohydrates.

Here is what you need to know:

In order for your body to use the energy that has been stored in a carbohydrate, it must be broken down into one of the more simple sugars (like glucose or fructose). When your body digests complex carbohydrates, it simply clips off one of the glucose molecule blocks and the glucose molecule enters the blood stream where it is used by the body. That is really all digestion entails for carbohydrates – cutting simple monosaccharides off larger groups of disaccharides, oligosaccharides, and polysaccharides.

The reason why your body wants to chop the large carbohydrate branches up into smaller glucose blocks is because glucose is your body's main energy source... its gasoline. While your body can convert every major source of food (fats, proteins, carbohydrates) into energy, its favorite, by far, is glucose. Your body's preference for glucose probably accounts, in part, for our craving for all sugar foods.

What you will notice about this process of clipping off single glucose molecules from larger chains is that it takes energy and time. Since removing glucose blocks from complex branches takes a while, your blood sugar will rise slowly whenever you are eating more complex carbohydrates. This is how your body is used to absorbing sugars – slowly over time (unless you choose to get your carbohydrates out of a soda can, in which case your blood sugar will rise rapidly). Whenever you drink a soda, you are getting some of the simplest carbohydrates on the planet (sucrose, fructose, or glucose) and these sugars are directly absorbed into your blood stream. No work at all is required by your body to absorb these sugars.

Remember this: The result of drinking a soda is a rapid rise in your blood sugar.

When carbohydrates are more complex (think oligosaccharide or polysaccharide), it takes some effort for your body to digest them. Whenever your body has to work to break off glucose or other sugars from long chains of carbohydrates, your blood sugar will rise much more slowly. This is why, say nutritionists, it is better to eat complex carbohydrates. The rise in your blood sugar happens over a longer period of time and does not reach the high peaks associated with consuming simple sugars.

By now you can probably identify which are the simple and which are the complex carbohydrates, but let's walk through an example of how, with the magic of processing, we can turn a complex carbohydrate into a simple carbohydrate.

Changing Complex into Simple

If you were to walk out into a farmer's field, grab some wheat seeds off of a stalk and start munching on them, you would find it very difficult to break down sugars in your raw-grain meal. You could probably chew the grain a bit and eventually swallow it, but it would take some effort on your part. If you ate a handful of these grains and took a blood sample, you would find that your blood sugar would rise very little, if at all. The reason your blood sugar wouldn't rise is simple: Grains straight from the field are about as complex of a carbohydrate as you can get. It is difficult for your body to break down and release the glucose molecules that are locked inside the polysaccharides that make up a wheat grain.

The first kind of processing we could try would also be the easiest. Let's throw the grain into a pot of water and boil it for a while. Boiling the grains have not changed them much, but your body now finds it easier to digest and easier to extract the simple sugars from the grain. If we checked your blood, we would find that your blood sugar has increased more than it did when eating the grain directly from the field, but not much more.

But, let's not stop there. What if we take the processing a little further by now grinding the grains. Grinding breaks down the fibers that hold the grain together and creates more surface area, this allows more digestion to take place. Grinding the grain means that your body is able to access the stored sugars easier. You would expect to see a larger rise in blood sugar when the grain is ground and eaten than when you try to eat grains straight from the field. If you cook this ground-up grain in some way, such as making porridge, you have made even more sugars available to your body. If you were to mix the whole grain with water, add yeast, and make whole wheat bread, you are, once again, making even more sugars available to your body.

There is still another processing step you could take to make even more sugars available to your body. If you were to remove much of the outer coating of the wheat grain (the bran and germ), and grind the inner grains, you would get something called white flour. Once you have removed the outer layers of the grain, your body has an even easier time getting to the sugars that are in the wheat grain. In fact, it is so easy to get to the sugars in white bread that your body can't tell the difference between eating table sugar or white bread. Eating white bread increases your blood sugar just as high as if you were eating white sugar.

Did you catch that, class? White bread and white sugar increase your blood sugar identically.

There you go: from complex carbohydrate to simple carbohydrate with one grain, all dependent upon how much you decide to process the grain.

Breads and processed grains are the so-called isocaloric starches that the American Diabetes Association was talking about in the introduction to this book. If you remember the quote from the association, it said that table sugar doesn't change our blood sugar more than eating isocaloric starches and they are right. White sugar acts just like white bread (or other isocaloric starches): Eat either of them and your blood sugar rises.

I will have much more to say about how foods change our blood sugar later in the book, but just know for now that the more complex the carbohydrate, the less it will make your blood sugar rise (and that is a good thing).

Not to stomp on all that you have just learned in your high school class, but for a long time we simply assumed that the more complex the carbohydrate, the less our blood sugar would rise. This assumption continued for many years until a brilliant scientist decided to examine what foods actually do in the human body and how they affect blood sugar. From this work, the Glycemic Index was born... a new way of looking at foods and how they affect blood sugar. What we found out from actually measuring blood sugar is that some complex carbohydrates act the way we thought they would and some don't.

The bell rings in the classroom and tells you that this science class has come to an end. While you may hope that you can now leave school for the day, why don't you take a trip down the hall to the history department? Let's take a peek at the history of sugar. Sugar's history is interesting and has a lot to teach us about how important sugar has become to humans.

The Rise of Sugar

The next time you are in a grocery store, pick up a bag of sugar and read the label. You will notice the label likely claims that the bag of sugar is 99 percent pure; this is what purity laws require in order for something to be called table sugar. What the bag is telling you though, now that we all remember our high school science lesson, is that it contains 99 percent sucrose. Table sugar used to contain sugar from sugar cane, but now it can contain sugar from cane or sugar beets. The end result is the same no matter what plant is used – a bag full of sucrose.

If we could again step back into that field some 10,000 years ago, you would be unable to find anything remotely similar to that bag of sucrose we find everywhere today. Nature simply does not create a concentrated sweet substance remotely resembling sugar.

You may stop me right here and say that honey is found in nature and is as sweet as sugar; I would have to agree with you on that point. But I would also point out that honey is a processed food, it is just the bees doing the processing rather than a modern manufacturing plant. The other point to be made about honey is to ask yourself: How much honey could you realistically gather in your lifetime if you couldn't find it on your grocery shelf? How many times a week would you want to battle with bees to be able to eat their honey? Since honey is not a realistic option, we can agree that concentrated sugar doesn't really exist in nature.

Much time and effort is required to make that bag of sugar in your grocery store. Let's take a look at where it all started.

Sweet History

From non-existence, to luxury, to being consumed in almost every meal… sugar has slowly crept into our diet. Remember, if you are typical, you eat around one-quarter to one-half a pound of sugar every day. Whether you know it or not, sugar makes up a large percentage of the calories you put in your mouth.

The history of sugar is fascinating and varied. It is a story that spans the globe, involves the slave trade, wars, money, power, and intrigue. There are entire books dedicated to the history of sugar and it is not my intention to delve into the entire story here, but to just give you a little taste (pun intended).

The origin of sugar is lost to time, but sugar cane, a tropical grass, probably originated in New Guinea. During prehistoric times sugar was grown and eventually spread throughout the Pacific Islands and into India. The first process for making sugar required squeezing the plant in a press and then evaporating off the water. The credit for developing this process goes to India and occurred somewhere around 500 BC. From these humble beginnings, sugar has taken the world by storm.

There are records of sugar arriving in China around 200 BC where the Chinese quickly added sugar cane to the plants they were cultivating. Western countries learned of sugar cane as a result of military expeditions to India and beyond. It is said that Nearchos, one of Alexander the Great's commanders, described sugar cane as "a reed that gives honey without bees." The real advancement in sugar production began in the Mediterranean regions of Sicily, Cyprus, Crete, and Malta around 600 AD. Large sugar plantations, factories, and the first sugar mills all started around this time and sugar use quickly spread to the rest of Europe.

Even though sugar was being processed and grown in many parts of the world at this time, it was still considered a luxury. While estimations of costs are hard to determine, it is generally accepted that by the year 1300, a pound of sugar was equal to a year's salary for most people in Europe. Needless to say, not too many people were using sugar to bake cookies back then.

As sugar gained in popularity, more land was needed to grow sugar cane. Parts of the African coast were well suited to grow the plant and this helped to spur the conquest and enslavement of much of Africa.

Sugar came to the New World in and around 1500 when it was discovered that many parts of the Caribbean were especially well suited to growing sugar cane. The need for sugar increased the need for land and manpower; this led to a frenzied take-over of lands and an increase in slave trade activity.

It is estimated that over five million slaves transported to the Americas during the eighteenth century were destined to work in the sugar cane fields or in related branches of the sugar industry. Imagine the cost (both in human suffering and monetarily) associated with the removal and transporting of millions of people from their homes in Africa and other parts of the world, all to support the world's growing sugar habit. Could sugar really be that important?

During the 1700s, the price of sugar began to drop, making the sweet stuff enormously popular. People began to change the way that they were eating. Jams, candy, and sweetened coffee and tea, along with other processed foods began to enter most people's lives around this time. The more sugar became a staple of daily life, the more land was cleared to raise sugar cane, leading to an explosion in sugar markets and sugar companies.

In 1747, a German chemist, Andreas Marggraf, discovered that sucrose (sugar) could be extracted from sugar beets. The discovery was ignored until 1813 when Napoleon, then at war and cut off from the Caribbean sugar supply by British war ships, ordered the planting of sugar beets to feed France's sugar addiction. Sugar from sugar beets now accounts for about thirty percent of the world sugar production.

From 1800 on, the amount of sugar consumption and production steadily increased. Sugar, while fairly common, was still rationed during World Wars I and II. The real drop in costs and the efficiency of production has occurred in the last fifty years or so. No longer does a pound of sugar cost a year's worth of wages. Today a pound of sugar can be bought for less than an hour's worth of work for most people: Cheap and readily available, the perfect combination for an addictive substance.

High Fructose Corn Syrup

The story of sugar wouldn't be complete without discussing the newest sugar on the block: high-fructose corn syrup (HFCS). High-fructose corn syrup comes, of course, from corn, but it takes a bit of processing for it to get from the field to your table and soda can.

High-fructose corn syrup is cheaper and sweeter than traditional sugars and is now replacing sucrose in many of our foods and beverages. The consumption of HFCS increased over one thousand percent between 1970 and 1990, it now accounts for about ten percent of all the calories consumed by a typical person. Think about it: Ten percent of your calories are likely to come from a single source: corn. This may seem impossible until you learn about all the foods that contain this sugar. HFCS can be found in soda, pancake syrup, candy, chips, ketchup, and more.

To make high-fructose corn syrup, manufacturers first process corn into a simple corn syrup that is mostly glucose. Manufacturers then use an enzymatic process to convert much of the glucose into fructose. To get HFCS, further processing is needed. The end result is that approximately half of the glucose is transformed into fructose.

When processed, HFCS is very similar to table sugar. Table sugar, or sucrose (remember?) is a disaccharide of glucose and fructose bonded together. HFCS, though, is a mixture of about forty-five percent glucose and fifty-five percent fructose. The problem with HFCS is that it contains a large amount of free fructose. Fructose is a unique sugar that is treated far differently in your body than glucose. Let's take a closer look.

Fructose and glucose are both simple sugars (monosaccharides). They are very similar in chemical structure. Fructose is known as "fruit sugar" because it is the main sugar found in fruits; it tastes about twice as sweet as sucrose (table sugar). Even though these sugars are almost identical on a molecular level, the digestion, absorption, and metabolism of fructose is very different from that of glucose. Fructose has long been recommended for people with diabetes because it does not lead to the same increase in the amount of sugar in your blood (blood sugar) as other sugars, but this distinction, as we shall see, is meaningless.

Your cells can use glucose directly, but when you consume fructose, your liver has to process the sugar before it can be used by your body.

The liver has basically two choices when fructose arrives to be processed. It can change the fructose into glucose, thereby enabling the cells of the body to use the sugar for energy, or the liver can convert the fructose into fat. Studies suggest that converting fructose into fat is what the liver prefers to do with this sugar.[1]

Some researchers believe that consuming large amounts of fructose is the real reason why we have seen such an explosion in the number of overweight and obese people throughout the world. The liver converting fructose into fat may also lead to high cholesterol, high triglycerides, insulin resistance (and eventually diabetes), and a host of other complications.[2] There is also evidence that this fructose fat-conversion may lead to a condition know as fatty liver.[3] Either way, having fructose converted into fat is not good for anyone.

The last thing you should know about fructose is what scientists mean when they say "blood sugar." You may know that your body controls the amount of sugar in your blood very tightly. When the body's sugar control mechanism fails, you have a condition called diabetes, which leads to large spikes in blood sugar. High blood sugar, as we will learn, can lead to a whole series of conditions that are likely to shorten the time you spend on earth.

The tool used to test the amount of sugar in your blood is called a glucometer (a glucose meter). At this point, armed with your high school science class lesson, you may be thinking, "Of course, if you had a glucose meter you wouldn't detect any fructose because they are two different sugars." And you'd be absolutely right. Your glucometer would not show a rise in blood sugar because you'd be measuring an entirely different sugar.

So why is it that doctors and scientists are not picking up on this vital distinction? If it's obvious to high school students that a glucometer can only measure glucose levels, why do medical professionals seem oblivious to this fact? Why is it that doctors and scientists think it is NOT okay to have a large rise in blood glucose (a sugar), and call that disease diabetes, but they insist on believing it IS okay to have a rise in blood fructose (another sugar)?

It seems an ironic twist of modern medicine that we have been testing blood sugar for years looking only at blood glucose when the real culprit (fructose) may have been completely ignored. The truth is that both glucose and fructose cause problems for different reasons, but thinking that fructose is somehow better than glucose is an illusion that must be forever shattered, especially those with diabetes.

Drinking Sugars

The last stop on our sugar tour is to try to understand what happens when we drink sugars. While this may sound as though it's straightforward, a sugar drink is not the same as a sugar food.

If your body is woefully unable to handle the processed sugars we eat every day, it is even less adept at handling those same sugars when you drink them. In the last twenty years, soda consumption has risen over 300 percent in the United States, causing a multitude of health problems.[4] Numerous scientific studies have demonstrated that the more soda you drink the more likely you are to be overweight.[5] Let's find out why.

Normally, when you put a food into your mouth you chew it. The simple act of chewing begins a series of events that alerts your body that it should expect nutrients and a rise in blood sugar. When you first put foods into your mouth and begin chewing, the stomach starts secreting stomach acid to prepare for the meal. Hormones are released when we begin to eat. Each of these hormones is designed to help your body deal with the rise in blood sugar that occurs whenever a food hits your stomach.

When you drink calories, something strange happens. The hormones normally released during a meal are not activated.[6] This is especially true when the calories are comprised of simple sugars. The other problem is that when you drink something that is very sweet, especially when you drink it outside of a meal, there is almost no digestion that takes place. This means that the sugar in the soda goes from the can directly into your blood stream.

It is as though your body does not understand calories in liquid form. Who could blame it? Ten thousand years ago, the only two liquids to be found on the entire planet were breast milk and water.

So imagine for a moment how confused your body must be when you drink a soda. Your body is just hanging out, minding its own business, and suddenly a large amount of sugar gets dumped into the blood stream. "What is going on?" your body thinks, "No one sent us a message that our blood sugar was going to rise." Nevertheless, the sugar needs to be taken care of somehow, so your body begins to process it.

Normally, when you are eating and hormones have been released, a hormone communicates to your brain that you are full and should stop eating. Because hormones haven't been released when you drink a soda, there is no message to your brain telling you that you should stop consuming food. This means that you are hungry and still eating, even though there is enough sugar-energy running around in your body to meet your needs.

All along I have been picking on soda, but the problems with soda are also true for fruit juices as well. Any sugar that enters your mouth in a liquid form is bound to create problems for you and your confused body. Drinking calories can lead to a weight-gaining triple-combination: Studies have shown that drinking sodas or fruit juices decreases insulin sensitivity, feelings of fullness, and can lead to overeating during the day.[7]

At this point you probably recognize the trouble you are in if the soda you are drinking happens to be made with fructose, such as high fructose corn syrup. When you drink something sweet, especially if it is fructose-sweetened, you don't feel full, you eat more, and your cells become insensitive to insulin. If you also consider the fact that your body easily turns fructose into fat, and that it has a hard time recognizing sugars when you drink them, and that sugar is addictive, you have the perfect recipe for obesity, diabetes, heart disease, and other major health problems. Maybe soda should come with a warning: Drink this product at your own risk.

You Did It!

Okay, you made it through your high school class and now have the tools you need to understand the rest of our journey through this book. The next two chapters deal with the addictive qualities of sugar and what happens when sugar enters your blood stream.

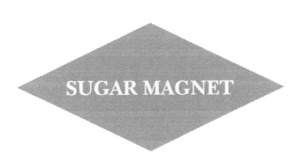

SUGAR MAGNET

Here is the question that may have been in the back of your mind the whole time you have been reading this book: Can sugar really be as addictive as cigarettes? To answer that question, let's first ask a few other questions.

When was the last time you gorged on a whole bag of broccoli? You saw the broccoli in the store, bought it, and started eating it on the way home and it was so good you ate it all before you made it through your front door. What about other vegetables or protein? Have you ever gorged yourself with steak, carrots, or green beans?

While it is not likely that you have gorged on any of those foods, I'm guessing you can remember multiple times when you sat down to eat only a few chips and then finished the entire bag. Or, maybe, you thought you would only have a few pieces of candy, but finished all that was in the house. Maybe the food you gorged on was ice cream, pretzels, bread, or chips, or some other carbohydrate. Have you ever baked cookies or other sweets and ate them until you felt sick? Feeling bad, though, didn't keep you from doing the very same thing the next day with the rest of what you baked.

Cravings can happen with any food and, yes, you may have cravings for broccoli, steak, apples, or green beans, but what is different about those cravings is that they are easily satisfied. Typically, you crave the food, eat it, and the craving ends. Carbohydrates are not like that. What is especially telling about binging on carbohydrates is that you may have binged on them even though you weren't hungry. The question that we need to answer is this: What makes carbohydrates so special?

Welcome to Your Addiction

Most grains and sugars share this defining characteristic: People binge on them. They binge on carbohydrates more than they do on any other type of food. I call it "the sugar magnet" – once you put any sugar or a food that acts like sugar into your mouth, more wants to follow.

To find out if you are addicted to sugar, let's first try running a little experiment in your mind. The people who can do this experiment best are people who have dieted, especially if their diet limited carbohydrates and sugars, as with the Atkins or South Beach diets. Think back to when you tried one of the diets; your diet probably followed a typical pattern.

First, you may have picked up a low-carbohydrate diet book or a friend told you how well the diet worked and you decided to give it a try. Not eating any grains or sugars sounded difficult, but you wanted to lose weight. You may have had a few false starts when you began the diet only to fall off it the same day. Or you managed to get going, but the diet lasted only a few days. Finally, you got tired of looking at yourself in the mirror and decided that you would, without fail, begin the diet. Either way, the first day of the diet was extremely difficult. You may have experienced headaches, shakiness, moodiness, and were quick to anger. After a few days on the diet, though, these symptoms disappeared and you began to feel much better. If you are typical, you had more energy, your sense of taste and smell improved, your digestion was better, and you may have even slept better. And wow! You began to lose weight – it really worked!

But then, the sugar magnet strikes again!

You may have been on the diet for a few weeks, a few months, or even as long as a year when a thought crept into your mind. The thought that danced in your head was the vision of a donut or a potato chip or (insert your favorite carbohydrate or sugary food here). You liked how you felt and looked on your new diet, but the craving for that food became irresistible. You tried to put the thought of (insert your favorite carbohydrate or sugary food here) out of your mind, but it kept coming back. Eventually, you said to yourself, "I'll just try a little bite; a little bit won't cause any harm."

The other way this may have happened is that you experienced an emotional upset: a bad day at work, a fight with a spouse or friend, money problems, or any number of tough issues. You began to seek comfort, believing you needed or deserved it because of what you were going through.

You decided to take a bite.

If the food you were craving was a sugary food, once it entered your mouth, you think, "Wow, that is sweet. I had no idea just how sweet that food was." We tend to adapt to the foods we are eating. It is only by staying away from them that we realize just how strong they are. Cigarette smokers and people who drink alcohol experience the same thing when they return to their addiction.

If you are like most people, when you tasted the food you were craving, it was okay, but not as great as you imagined it was going to be. You may have wondered why you were craving it in the first place, but you ate it all anyway. Eating this snack also probably didn't have the effect you thought it would. In fact, you may have felt worse than you did before you took a bite. You then swore that you would never eat that food again. But within an hour or two, here comes the sugar magnet, and you suddenly wanted that sugar food again. Soon you were binging again on any carbohydrate foods you could find.

This is typically how the whole diet disintegrates. All it took was one bite and that was the end of your diet, your weight loss, and how good you felt. Once those carbohydrates hit your mouth, you were back to eating the same, or worse, than you did before. Many people are left thinking about how awful they are for not being able to control themselves.

Sound familiar?

Consider what you've just read. How did I know that something like this had probably happened to you? Because what I just described happens to everyone; well, it happens to everyone who has an addiction to carbohydrates. Every person reading this book who has tried a low carbohydrate diet will recognize their own series of events in what I've just described...events that are all eerily similar.

Now take a moment to re-read the paragraphs above, but instead of your favorite carbohydrate or sugary food, insert any other addicting substance: cigarettes, alcohol, or any addicting drug. The story is the same for all addicts. At first, quitting an addiction is very difficult. Once a habit is kicked, the person experiences withdrawal symptoms. After a period of time, people tend to feel better, but, if the addicting substance is ever tried again, it typically leads to binging, often in greater quantities than before.

Have you ever wondered why so many people lose weight only to gain back more than they lost? Being addicted to a substance and removing it will always cause binging when the addictive substance is re-introduced. And when we are talking about sugar, the binging results in weight gain.

Evidence

Most people, when they think about the above "experiment," are convinced that sugars and foods that act like sugar in their body are addictive. But let's consider what the scientific community has to say about the sugar-addiction connection.

The evidence for the addictive qualities of sugar comes primarily from animal studies. There are ways to study addiction in people, but the studies simply have not been done. Another reason we have limited studies on human beings is likely because most scientists do not consider the possibility that sugar may be addictive...they simply assume that it isn't.

Before we learn what scientific studies have been done, let's revisit the sugar industry website and see what they have to say about sugar addiction:

> ### Is Sugar Addictive?
> *Addiction is compulsive behavior with medically identifiable physiological symptoms. Eating sugar or any other carbohydrate (or proteins or fats) does not produce these symptoms. The premise put forth by some (not the consensus of the scientific community) is the pleasure*

one experiences from eating food causes changes in brain chemistry that lead to addiction. It is well known that all pleasurable experiences (one good example is exercise) generate chemical responses in the brain, but all changes in neurochemistry do not equate to addiction. The science on food addiction is limited and most of that science has been conducted with rats.

The reality is people like tasty foods. But there are distinct differences between a psychological dependency that is often an emotional response to food and actual physical dependence. Food does not generate withdrawal, the medically distinct symptoms characteristic of authentic addiction.[1]

The sugar industry seems proud to point out that only a few studies concerning sugar and addiction have been done and most of these have been conducted on rats. This is not true. As you shall see, there are actually quite a lot of animal studies on sugar addiction. While sugar addiction hasn't been studied much in human beings, there is certainly evidence that sugar dependency – whether psychological or physical – is indeed an addiction. An addiction that is similar to every other acknowledged addiction. And what the sugar industry fails to point out is that there are no studies that show the opposite: That sugar is *not* addictive. Every time sugar is tested, it has been shown to be addictive.

Perhaps sugar addiction hasn't been studied extensively in human beings because few scientists have asked the question, "Is it a real addiction?" They assume, maybe because they haven't taken a trip in a time machine like we have, that the way we are eating today is exactly the way we have always eaten. Remember, no one questions the wearing of shoes because so many people wear them.

Addictions

Let's look at addiction in general. At this point, it doesn't matter if we are talking about cigarettes, alcohol, or other hard drugs. To be sure, every addiction has their own unique features, but most people with addictions act surprisingly similar.

If an addict tries to quit, they generally go through these stages:

- **Stage one: Deciding to quit**. Denial is actually a common first stage, but why don't we assume that the addict has come to the realization that they need to change? The addict acknowledges that their smoking, drinking, or drug use is uncontrollable and there is a strong need for change. A typical addict will decide to quit multiple times before actually following through. They often say to themselves, "Tomorrow is the last day that I will smoke," and yet, they wake up the next morning and begin smoking again. They will often go through this routine numerous times before making an actual change. Occasionally people do decide to quit quickly and this is often spurred on by a traumatic event that makes them realize that their addiction is a problem.

- **Stage Two: Quitting**. Here, an addict will actually make it to the stage where they get rid of their drug of choice and make an effort to stop using it. When they do this, their body rebels: headaches, tremors, mood swings, sweats, and sometimes even life-threatening symptoms can be associated with removing the addiction.

- **Stage Three: Improvement**. In this stage, people are feeling better. They may still want their drug, but are now seeing clearer, feeling more energized, sleeping better, and are in a much better mood.

- **Stage Four: Temptation**. Addicts are always tempted, but they will try to keep their temptation under control. They often begin to believe that they have so much control that they imagine they will be able to return to using the drug without going overboard. But as soon as they decide to try their addiction just once, they discover how little control they have and begin binging on their addiction. In fact, a key sign of addiction is that removal of the substance causes an overuse once they start using again.

Does any of this sound at all familiar? Perhaps it sounds exactly like the last time you went on a diet. If you have ever tried a sugarless and carbohyrateless diet, all of this will seem painfully familiar.

The value in viewing sugar as an addiction is that doing so helps to put into perspective so many of the problems that people run into when trying to lose weight. The craving and the binging all become understandable when you see sugar foods as addictive. People try, but they just can't shake their cravings.

Remember that with most addictions, people need more and more of what they are addicted to in order to feel the same effects. This is why people constantly gain more weight after they go on a diet, despite how they feel or what the addiction is doing to their body. Compulsive use of a substance without regard for the negative consequences is another common theme in people with addictions.

Let's stop here and take a look at the studies that are available and see what happens when rats and sugar are combined.

Rat Addicts

Rats like sugar. In fact, most animals, when given a choice, will choose sugar over most any food. While the sugar industry is correct when saying there are limited studies on the addictive properties of sugar, the studies that have been done are dramatic.

Here are summaries from various studies examining the effects of sugar on rats:

> Rats that were given sugar occasionally and then allowed to eat as much as they desired, binged on the sugar. The ingestion of sugar caused changes in their brains similar to rats that were addicted to morphine-like drugs. The researchers noted that there were some minor differences between the brains of opiate-addicted (codeine, morphine, and heroin are opioid drugs) rats and sugar-addicted rats, but overall the brain response was similar.[2]
>
> *-Brain Research. Molecular Brain Research*, **2004**

> Rats given sugar were much more likely to gain weight and eat more calories than rats that didn't eat sugar. When the sugar was removed from their diet, they showed signs of withdrawal similar to the effects of withdrawal from other drugs, such as alcohol, nicotine, and opiates.[3]
>
> *- Nutritional Neuroscience*, **2005**

Researchers in this review study suggest there is a close link between opiates and sugar. Taking opioids leads to an increase in sugar craving. Eating sugar causes a release of natural opioids in the body, stimulating more sugar craving. This is what is called a feed-forward cycle: doing *something* causes more of that *something* to happen. In this case, eating sugar leads to more sugar eating; otherwise known as the sugar magnet.[4]

- Lakartidninge, 2005

The researchers in this study confirm that the consumption of sugar shows all the signs of addiction. When rats are given sugar over a long period of time, and then have the sugar removed, they show signs of withdrawal that any junkie would recognize: teeth chattering, forepaw tremors, and head shaking. When the rats were given sugar again, they binge, eating increasingly larger amounts of sugar. One way to know if someone is addicted to opioids is to give them a drug, such as Naloxone, that blocks the opioids in the brain. When Naloxone, for example, is given to drug addicts, they experience withdrawal symptoms. Giving Naloxone to sugar-addicted rats produces the exact same withdrawal symptoms, suggesting that sugar affects their brains similar to the way in which other opioid-like drugs do.[5]

- Obesity Research, 2002

This study showed that when rats have sugar available in their cages, they eat more (up to thirty-five percent) rat chow than rats with no access to sugar. Sugar, this study suggests, may cause an increase in the number of calories consumed in a day. Interestingly, removing sugar from the rats made them more likely to bite and be aggressive.[6]

-Psychological Reports, 2002

Use of drugs of addiction is often increased during times of stress. When people feel stressed out, they turn to their addiction for comfort. The researchers in this study demonstrated a link between sugar-addicted rats and their increased use of sugar following a stressful event.[7]

- *Psychopharmacology*, **2000**

This study also confirmed the stress-sugar response. Stress may induce bursts of binge eating or drug addiction relapse. Researchers suggest it may be due to a brain chemical called corticotropin-releasing factor (CRF).[8]

- **BMC Biology, 2006**

Sugar addicted rats in this study were shown to have delayed satiation response, meaning that it took them longer to feel full and stop eating than non-sugar-addicted rats. These rats also release more dopamine in their brains than non-addicted animals; this is the exact response seen in other drug-addicted brains.[9]

- *Neuroscience*, **2005**

Researchers in this study wanted to find out what would happen to the brains of sugar-addicted rats if they removed sugar from the rats' diets for two weeks. When they examined the rats' brains, even after weeks without any sugar, they still had the same brain changes seen in addicts. This study supports what many addicts say: "Once an addict, always an addict." It does not matter whether they are taking the drug or not.[10]

- *Physiology & Behavior*, **2005**

Another study shows that intermittent, excessive sugar intake causes changes in brain receptors of rats similar to the alterations brought on by the ingestion of other drugs of abuse.[11]

- *Neuroreport*, **2001**

This study conducted on human beings highlighted the way in which sugar and alcoholism are related. The researchers found that people who are alcoholics were more likely to gain weight and have a preference for sweet foods.[12]

- *Addictive Behaviors*, 2006

The sugar-addicted rats in this study had all foods taken away from them. They experienced drug-like withdrawal symptoms including anxiety and brain changes such as dopamine and acetylcholine imbalance. The researchers suggest that this addictive process may be part of the reason for some eating disorders, such as bulimia or binging and purging.[13]

- *Physiology & Behavior*, 2008

In an interesting study, when given a choice, rats actually preferred sugar over cocaine. In spite of the fact that cocaine is one of the most addictive drugs, the rats would shun cocaine in favor of sugar.[14]

- *PLoS ONE*, 2007

The following are a collection of reviews, which are a gathering of many studies together in one place, in order to comment on trends in research. They generally are more respected than a single clinical study.

Researchers in this review confirm that sugar addiction is similar to other addictions including binging, withdrawal symptoms, increased intake following removal of the addiction (abstinence), and cross-sensitization (addiction to sugar and other substances of abuse). Brain changes similar to those found in addicts of other drugs of abuse also occur in sugar-addicts.[15]

- *Experimental and Clinical Psychopharmacology*, 2007

This review, entitled "Of human bondage: food craving, obsession, compulsion, and addiction," confirms that drug addiction and sugar addiction share many common features.[16]

-*Physiology & Behavior*, **2002**

This review suggests the link between sugar consumption and alcoholism is real, noting that people who have a preference for sweet tastes also are more likely to become alcoholics.[17]

- *Alcohol and Alcoholism*, **1999**

This review of many studies examines the possibility that sugar is an addictive substance. It suggests that sugar addiction is possible given that sugar releases opioids and dopamine in the brain, both of which have the potential to be addictive. Sugar consumption has been paired with binging, withdrawal, craving, and cross-sensitization. These behaviors have been associated with neurochemical changes in the brain that occur as a result of the ingestion of addictive drugs.[18]

- *Neuroscience and Biobehavioral reviews*, **2008**

A Summary of Research on Rat Addicts

As you can see, there is actually a lot of research on the subject of sugar addiction. The rats in these studies have a lot to teach us. Let me sum it up for you:

- When rats have free access to sugar, they will eat a ton of it and will eat more sugar than any other food available to them.
- When sugar is removed from the diet of rats that have become used to it, they shake, tremble, are anxious, and their teeth chatter. They are also prone to aggression. Any addict or junkie will recognize these classic withdrawal symptoms.

- When sugar is removed from the diet of rats and when sugar is returned to their diet, rats will binge on the sugar. Similar to alcoholism and other addictions, this "deprivation-effect" is a phenomenon that explains what happens when the removal of a substance for a period of time results in an increased use of the substance and uncontrollable cravings upon its return.

- When under stress, rats will consume more sugar.

- When scientists look into the brains of rats, they find that there are physical changes along with increases in brain chemicals that are very similar to those of other addicts including alcoholics, smokers, and opioid users.

- One of the best ways to study if a substance you are taking is addictive is to inject what is called an opioid antagonist. When animals raised on excessive intake of sugar are given such a drug, they experience anxiety and other signs of withdrawal similar to morphine or nicotine withdrawal. When scientists give sugar to rats for a long period of time and give them a drug (Naloxone) that actually blocks the brain from experiencing brain chemicals associated with drug abuse, the rats experience all the symptoms of withdrawal.

- Cross-sensitization exists with sugar addiction. In other words, when someone is addicted to sugar, they have a greater risk of being addicted to alcohol, nicotine, and morphine-like drugs.

While it is true that many more studies, especially human studies, need to be done, the medical community cannot ignore that sugar has addictive qualities. These studies are far from insignificant as the sugar industry would have you believe. There are good reasons to believe that sugar is an addiction every bit as powerful as any other addiction.

Sugar as a Gateway Drug?

Some of the most intriguing studies about sugar addiction are those suggesting that sugar addiction may lead to other addictions. We give sugar to young children; we give and take sugar to modify our moods; we give and take sugar as a reward. If we are convinced by the rat studies highlighting the physical changes that occur in our brains and bodies that compel us to eat sugar in ever increasing amounts, it is no wonder that some of us will seek out even higher highs.

While the current evidence that sugar is a gateway drug leading to other addictions is minimal, it does provide some "food" for thought.

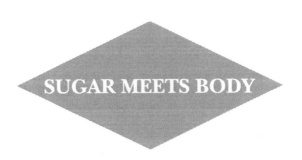

SUGAR MEETS BODY

Sugar addiction, by itself, is really not a problem. Well... it wouldn't be a problem if sugar wasn't also harmful. After all, if cigarettes were addictive, but they made you live longer, removed grey hair, and made your breath smell great, everyone would be happy with their addiction. Cigarettes, of course, do cause harm and the harm is not just to the smoker's lungs; they also increase the risk of heart disease, stroke, and any number of cancers including lung, breast, bladder, and others. Sugar is the same; it increases the risk for many diseases.

It is actually easier than you would think to prove that sugar causes harm because we have a large population of people, diabetics, who are "experimenting" by having blood sugar much higher than the rest of the population. We can see the results of these "experiments" by watching which diseases develop in people who are diabetic. Sugar, it turns out, mimics cigarettes by causing harm, not just to teeth, but to multiple body systems.

Sugar causes harm through two mechanisms. The first is caused by having a high-octane fuel like sugar circulating in your arteries and veins. Just like cigarette smoke is harmful when it touches lungs, sugar is harmful when it touches blood vessels. This is what some researchers call the "toxic effect" of sugar; it damages the blood vessels that carry it throughout the body.

This damage, as we shall see, has far reaching consequences for your body and your health.

Sugar also causes harm because your body has to adjust to the high amount of sugar in the blood stream that occurs when you consume sugar foods. As your body attempts to control your blood sugar, it makes choices. These choices seem to work in the short term, but they often end up creating larger problems in the end. The sugar control mechanisms in your body start to falter and may eventually fail. Let's look at your body's sugar control mechanism and how it fails when you are eating high-octane sugar foods. We will later see how sugar and blood vessels shouldn't mix.

Welcome to the Sugar Coaster

Remember that many of the sugar foods we eat are rare in nature. Your body is simply not prepared to deal with such a large influx of sugar on a regular basis. As soon as you decide to drink that soda or eat that cake, you are off on a ride I like to call the sugar coaster. Once you are on the sugar roller coaster you are in for quite a ride!

There is typically a rush when you first eat something sugary and, of course, with a high comes the inevitable crash. We have all experienced a sugar crash: that awful feeling of tiredness following a sugar high. While a sugar high followed by a sugar crash is a common enough experience, the medical community has almost nothing to say about it. Some research papers talk about so-called "reactive hypoglycemia," but the well known sugar coaster doesn't register on scientific radar. This is probably because there is no way to measure your crash. If you were to measure someone's blood when they are experiencing a crash, in most cases you would find a normal blood sugar reading, so it is understandable that the medical community insists that nothing is wrong.

All test results are normal, yet you feel awful. What is going on?

The sugar crash may be the result of hormones that are released when you have a high amount of sugar in your body. Or it may be the result of how quickly your blood sugar drops, so while all appears normal, it is not. A sugar crash is probably the result of your body trying to rebalance after a surge in blood sugar. While the sugar crash remains a bit of a medical mystery, much more is known about how, over time, consuming a large amount of sugar does damage to your body's sugar control mechanism. Before we get there, let's first understand how your body controls blood sugar.

The Battle for Sugar Control

If you are typical, twenty percent of the calories you eat come from sugar.[1] That is a lot of calories that your body has to deal with that are pure white sugar and high fructose corn syrup. The control of sugar in your blood stream leads to a war of sorts between the sugar that you eat and your body's attempts to keep that blood sugar under control. This battle involves three players: the sugar you just ate, insulin (the main hormone used to control high blood sugar), and the cells in your body.

It is very important to your health to keep your blood sugar within a narrow range: not too high and not too low. To keep the sugar in your blood at a steady state, your body uses hormones. The most important hormone to reduce blood sugar is insulin. The body adjusts the amount of the insulin to the amount of sugar circulating in the blood. Low sugar in the blood means a low amount of insulin; high sugar means a high amount of insulin. Since we are all eating high sugar foods, this leads to a high amount of insulin in our bodies after each sugary meal. This high insulin level sets off a series of events that can move you away from efficient blood sugar control to poor blood sugar control and, of course, eventually to really bad blood sugar control, known as diabetes.

While the lifetime risk of developing diabetes is around thirty-two percent for males and thirty-eight percent for females[2] (higher in certain ethnic groups, such as Hispanic, Native American), many more people are in a pre-diabetic state or a syndrome called metabolic syndrome. Conservative estimates suggest approximately forty to fifty percent of the population are at risk of having either diabetes or metabolic syndrome. Those are pretty high risks.

People who are pre-diabetic or who have metabolic syndrome are beginning to lose blood sugar control. This uncontrolled blood sugar leads to two things: more uncontrolled blood sugar and widespread destruction of blood vessels in the body. Poor blood sugar control eventually leads to conditions such as diabetes, heart disease, stroke and others. Since approximately one-third of the people reading this book will eventually get diabetes, it is important to remember that having diabetes greatly reduces life expectancy. An individual diagnosed with diabetes at forty years of age will typically have his life shortened by nearly twelve years or her life shortened by fourteen years.[3] Having just metabolic syndrome will also cut years from your life expectancy.[4]

The Story of Insulin

Your body controls a lot of what goes on inside it with hormones – sugar control is no exception. Your body needs a way to control the amount of sugar in your blood and it needs to get that sugar from the blood vessels into the cells where it is used to produce energy. Glucagon, growth hormone, and catecholamines are hormones that raise blood sugar, while insulin is the hormone used to decrease blood sugar.

Let's focus on insulin. To understand how insulin and sugar interact, we have to visit a single cell in your body. Later we will look at the whole body because that is where the sugar and insulin story gets really interesting.

First we must look at where sugar is needed in the body.

Imagine that this is a cell in your body:

This could be a heart, muscle, brain, or any of the ten trillion cells in your body. The cell performs its cell functions and works as part of a whole to keep you alive and healthy.

All cells in your body control what enters or exits the cell. Cells use a sort of doorway system to control what goes in or what goes out. On the outside of the cell is a specialized structure called a receptor; receptors function as the doorway to the cell. There are receptors for all sorts of things that a cell may need and each receptor only opens its door for a specific hormone.

Let's say that typical receptors look like this:

There are receptors for all sorts of chemicals in your body, but imagine that the particular receptor we are looking at is for insulin. When the hormone insulin attaches to the receptor, the cell "opens up," and allows sugar enter the cell. Without these receptors, no sugar would get in.

So, a typical cell with insulin receptors would look like this:

Your body likes your blood sugar level to remain within a tight range. Doctors can measure blood sugar easily and when they do they find that your body tries to keep blood sugar levels between 70 and 140 mg/dL. Your blood sugar increases after eating sugar foods and your body will release insulin in an attempt to keep your blood sugar from going over the 140 mg/dL level. Healthy blood sugar control, in my opinion, would be keeping your blood sugar below 110 mg/dL. When the sugar in your blood starts to rise, your body senses this and secretes insulin.

Insulin, in our example, will look like this:

So, the process goes like this: As blood sugar rises, insulin is secreted, insulin travels to the cell and tells the cell to take up the sugar, blood sugar falls as the sugar enters the cells of the body and insulin is reduced. Simple enough, right?

Let's look at that in action inside our cell: Insulin connects to the receptor as shown in this image, telling the cell to open up, and letting sugar from the blood stream into the cell.

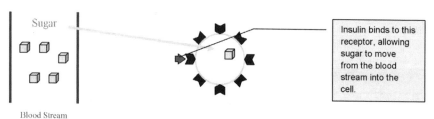

Sugar

Blood Stream

Insulin binds to this receptor, allowing sugar to move from the blood stream into the cell.

Pretty neat, huh?

At this point, everything is good. When insulin is released, the cells in the body fill up with sugar. Sugar is taken out of the blood stream, which, in turn, shuts off insulin secretion (remember that high blood sugar is what turns on insulin and when all the cells absorb the sugar, the amount of sugar in the blood drops and insulin gets turned off). Everybody is happy; the cells get the sugar energy they need, and the blood sugar is controlled within the range that the body likes.

All of this is a bit complicated, but let's keep going to see what happens when this blood sugar control mechanism starts to fail.

The Effects of High Blood Sugar

The story of how blood sugar goes into the cells is fairly unspectacular: blood sugar goes up, insulin goes up, sugar goes into the cells, blood sugar goes down, and insulin goes down. At least this is an unspectacular story unless the blood sugar becomes very high or the high-blood-sugar-dance continues for days and days.

If you eat food in the way that nature presents it to you, say a carrot, apple, or even rice and beans, you will find that both your blood sugar and insulin increase slowly.

A typical insulin response to a low carbohydrate meal would look like this: ➡ ➡ ➡

When you eat something containing a lot of sugar, say a soda, a cookie, or something sweet, the amount of insulin looks more like this: ➡➡➡➡➡➡➡

On the surface, this wouldn't appear to present a problem: more sugar, more insulin, so what's the big deal? The problem occurs back at the cell and what happens when this high amount of blood sugar occurs every day.

Let's take a look:

You just drank a soda, and here at the cell lots of insulin is telling the cell to take on more sugar:

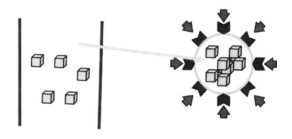

As you can imagine, there is only so much sugar any cell can handle. At a certain point the cell has enough sugar and doesn't want any more, but here is the problem: The cells in your body don't have an off switch.

Your body is woefully unprepared to handle high sugar and, therefore, there is no shut-off valve for cells that have too much sugar. If there is a large amount of insulin and sugar circulating in the body, the cells are obligated to take on all that sugar. This puts the cells of your body at a disadvantage, because too much sugar is harmful to the cell. Actually, your cells do have an option when faced with a large amount of sugar and insulin, but taking that option is a devil's bargain: It solves the problem for the individual cells, but creates a whole body disaster.

The Long-Term Effects of High Blood Sugar

If your blood sugar shoots up high occasionally, there is really no problem. The problem comes when your blood sugar is high over a long period of time or high blood sugar happens every day.

The cells in your body only want so much sugar; they just want enough sugar to do their jobs. When there is constantly too much insulin and too much sugar in the blood stream, the only response that the cells have is to remove the doorways (receptors) from the outside of the cell. This process is called down-regulation of receptors. When insulin receptors disappear throughout the body, it creates a whole-body effect called "insulin resistance," meaning the cells of the body become "resistant" to insulin.

Let's take a look at what happens to the cell when the body removes receptors:

A cell goes from having this many receptors:

To having, say, this many:

Now, this is a bit tricky to understand, but imagine if *all* the cells in your body began to respond to too much sugar by removing their insulin receptors. If every cell in the body removed its receptors (the doorways to sugar) what would happen? The end result would be that you'd have more sugar in your blood.

Why?

Remember that insulin used to be able to push sugar out of the blood stream and put it into the cells. The cells, though, are now getting rid of receptors because there is too much sugar around most of the time. The cells are becoming resistant to insulin. So, even though there is sugar in the blood stream and a lot of insulin, the sugar has no where to go because the cells won't allow it in. So, now, where does the sugar go? It stays in the blood stream.

But you also have to remember, more sugar in the blood stream creates what? The answer is more sugar in the blood stream leads to more insulin. When your body becomes insulin resistant, the next time you eat a meal, you have a higher amount of sugar in your blood because the cells are refusing to take on that sugar. So, more sugar in the blood stream means that the body will now release more insulin. Do you see the vicious cycle that is starting to develop? More insulin circulating in the body will eventually lead to fewer receptors on cells, which will lead to more sugar in the blood, and more insulin, and fewer receptors and…you get the idea.

Cells will eventually look like this as they get rid of even more receptors:

Now you understand how insulin resistance can develop from eating a high amount of sugar every day. The association between eating sugars and the creation of insulin resistance is, however, far from being a proven phenomenon in human beings. Animal studies demonstrate a relationship between eating sugars and foods that act like sugar and the development of insulin resistance,[5,6] but the medical community is far from convinced. Like much of the scientific study on sugar and health, much more research is needed.

Over Time

Okay. Let's see if we can pull this all together. Watch what happens over time, not to the individual cell, but in the whole body. The following chart shows how blood sugar and insulin react to each other and how insulin resistance builds over time when you are consuming sugar foods.

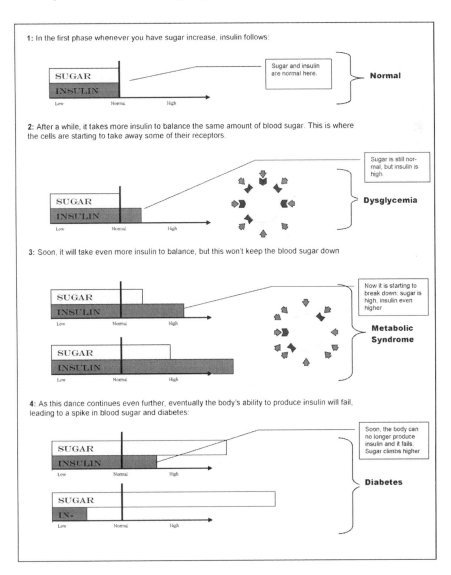

What happens over time with insulin resistance is that the body can no longer produce enough insulin and, eventually, insulin production fails. When the body can no longer produce enough insulin or the cells have become resistant to insulin, your body is no longer able to keep blood sugar within a narrow range. This is called diabetes, a situation where the blood sugar is very high.

But why is high sugar in the blood such a big deal? On the surface, high blood sugar doesn't really seem to be a problem. It actually is a problem and we will look closer at that in a moment. First, though, let's see what happens when your body can no longer stuff the cells of your body with sugar; after all, the sugar has to go somewhere.

What to Do with the Extra Sugar

After the cells have stopped taking on so much sugar, the body has to resort to other methods to dispose of the excess sugar.

In diabetics, that extra sugar may be dumped into their urine. Doctors can tell if a person is diabetic by testing the blood and urine for sugar. But even before a person becomes diabetic and begins dumping sugar into their blood and urine, the body has other ways to deal with the excess sugar.

To understand where the body is going to put the sugar, you have to understand what happens when you get hungry. Your appetite and feelings of hunger are controlled (no surprise) by hormones. When you haven't eaten in a while, your stomach starts producing a hormone called ghrelin. This hormone travels from your stomach to your brain and tells you that you are hungry. When you are hungry, generally you do what you are supposed to do: you eat. When you eat, your blood sugar and insulin increase; this, in turn, causes the release of another hormone found in fatty tissue, called leptin. Leptin travels to your brain and tells you that you are full. There are actually many more hormones involved in this dance, but this is basically the way it works: Ghrelin goes up, you feel hungry, you eat, and blood sugar and insulin go up, causing leptin to be released and you feel full and satisfied. This all changes when cells become insulin resistant.

As insulin resistance begins to set in, this whole system turns on its head and starts working against you, in the opposite way it was intended to work. High amounts of insulin actually block leptin from being released. This means that you have high blood sugar and high insulin and you still feel hungry. Normally, high blood sugar would mean that you are beginning to feel full. This broken mechanism may be, in part, responsible for overeating.

Things, however, get much worse for the person who has become insulin resistant. Insulin resistance forces the body to store more sugar and it stores much of this sugar as fat. For thousands of years, human beings have experienced times during which food was easily available and times when there was no food. So, what is the smartest thing to do with extra sugar? Store it. The fat cells of your body have a seemingly endless ability to store the excess sugar as fat. The problems with storing sugar as fat are many, but one of the most harmful is that more fat on your body means *more* insulin resistance. Here we go with another vicious cycle! Insulin resistance creates fat and weight gain, which leads to more insulin resistance and more fat gain and so on and so on. Unfortunately, the human body is perfectly designed to accommodate this vicious and incredibly unhealthy cycle.

Let's listen to a researcher who explains this hormonal cycle in a more technical way in a research article:

> *A thin, insulin-sensitive, 13-year-old boy might consume a daily allotment of 2,000 kcal, and burn 2,000 kcal daily in order to remain weight-stable, with a stable leptin level.*

> *However, if that same 13-year-old became hyperinsulinemic [high insulin] and/or insulin resistant, perhaps as many as 250 kcal of the daily allotment would be shunted to storage in adipose (fat) tissue, promoting a persistent obligate weight gain. Due to the obligate energy storage, he now only has 1,750 kcal per day to burn. The hyperinsulinemia [high insulin] also results in a lower level of leptin signal transduction, conveying a CNS (brain) signal of energy insufficiency. The remaining calories available are lower than his energy expenditure; the CNS [brain] would sense starvation. Through decreased SNS tone, he would reduce his physical activity, resulting in decreased quality of life; and through increased vagal tone, he would increase caloric intake and insulin secretion, but now at a much higher level.[7]*

In other words, insulin resistance not only causes more calories to be turned into fat, but it also makes the person experiencing insulin resistance feel hungry, even when they are eating the same amount of calories they were before they became insulin resistant.

Here it is again just to make sure you got it: As we become insulin resistant, not only do more of our calories get turned into fat, but we also feel hungry even when we have just eaten. And to make matters much worse, it is fructose that makes the conversion from blood sugar to fat much easier than glucose. This, of course, leads to insulin resistance even faster.[8]

Okay, now that we understand sugar control and how it can fail, let's look at the toxic effects of sugar on our blood vessels.

Sugar Destruction

People don't really die from diabetes because of the sugar running around in their blood. The body seems to be able to handle high blood sugar well enough, at least in the short term. In fact, you can have a very large amount of sugar running around in your blood and not even know it except for the fact that you have to go to the bathroom all the time. What really hurts people with diabetes is that sugar in the blood exerts a toxic effect on vital parts of the body.

In another not-thinking-the-next-thought-problem, doctors and scientists fully know what happens when blood sugar is high for too long in a diabetic. But they don't stop to think what happens when people who are pre-diabetic or seemingly normal consume large amounts of sugar. It is sort of like knowing that gasoline is deadly when you drink a lot of it, but somehow okay when you just sip it.

Most people are aware that diabetics are at risk of other diseases, they have more kidney disease, heart disease, stroke, numbness in their feet and hands, visual problems, and circulation disorders which can cause the loss of limbs. All of these health problems are caused by the toxic effects of a large amount of sugar circulating in the blood vessels.

Sugar Meets Blood Vessels

Sugar in high amounts is toxic to the body, especially to its blood vessels. Your body is crisscrossed with blood vessels; they provide the three most important things all your cells need: oxygen, nutrients, and energy. The blood vessels most vulnerable to sugar are the smaller ones, such as those in your eyes and kidneys, but it is becoming increasingly clear that sugar also damages the larger blood vessels (such as arteries and veins).

When sugar attacks blood vessels to such an extent that they stop working well, the cells that rely on that blood supply begin to fail. We can see this sugar destruction when we look at the diseases common among diabetics:

- **Atherosclerosis** (clogged arteries)
- **Nephropathy** (kidney damage)
- **Neuropathy** (nerve damage)
- **Retinopathy** (eye damage)

The link between all of these diseases is damaged blood vessels. To learn how sugar actually *becomes* toxic in your body, we have to return to our examination of the cells of the body.

At this point, I have to tell you that I didn't tell you the whole truth when I told you the story about the cells in your body, its receptors, and hormones. There are some cells that don't work by using the insulin receptor/doors to get sugar inside of them. These cells are called insulin-independent cells; they simply accept all the sugar that comes their way. While this might seem like an advantage, it actually isn't. When there is a high amount of sugar in the blood stream, there is also a high amount of sugar inside these insulin-independent cells, even when they don't need more sugar. These cells pay the price for having this open doorway to the blood stream when blood sugar is very high (as in someone with diabetes).

Do you want to guess where in the body these insulin-independent cells are?

If you look again at all the diseases that can be caused by high blood sugar, you have your answer: the blood vessels of the kidneys, eyes, and nerves. These tiny blood vessels, also called the microvasculature, are highly susceptible to the toxic effects of sugar.

Microvasculature

The cells of the tiny blood vessels in your body (microvasculature) cannot regulate the amount of sugar they allow inside and are damaged when the blood sugar is high and remains high for a long time. While scientists are all in agreement that these small blood vessel cells are harmed by sugar, the exact way in which the sugar harms them is still debatable. Currently, there are three competing ideas:[9]

1. Activation of the aldose-reductase pathway, leading to toxic accumulation of sorbitol.
2. Accelerated nonenzymatic glycosylation with deposition of advanced glycosylated end products (AGEs).
3. Activation of isoform(s) of protein kinase C (PKC) in vascular tissue, initiating a cascade of events culminating in diabetic complications.

All this gobbledegook really means is that the cells are overwhelmed by the amount of sugar inside of them and somehow must deal with the surplus sugar. In the end, the sugar either becomes something that is immediately harmful to the cell or, during the processing of sugar, cell-damaging free radicals form. Free radical damage is a bit complex, but most people have heard of the opposite of free radicals which are called antioxidants. The reason people take antioxidants is to stop free radical damage, but even taking a large amount of antioxidants won't help when a large amount of sugar is continually coursing through the blood stream.

Damage to the small blood vessels means that the vital parts of the body containing these blood vessels do not get sufficient nutrients; consequently, the cells being fed by these blood vessels begin to die. For example, the kidneys won't do their job as well and will begin dumping protein into the urine. The kidneys also play a role in maintaining blood pressure so when they are damaged, high blood pressure may result.

The cells of the eyes begin also begin to fail when exposed to high sugar. Eventually this damage can cause parts of the visual fields to go black. The eyes will attempt to fix the problem by growing new blood vessels, but this *fix* eventually blocks the visual fields, leading to blindness. When deprived of nutrients from blood vessels, the nerves throughout the body simply stop working and/or die. This can lead to numbness and sometimes to the pain and itching in the arm and legs that is common in diabetics.

While there are competing theories on why blood vessels become damaged, let's take a look at the most well-researched reason for their destruction: protein glycation, which can further change into advanced glycosylated end products (AGEs).

Protein Glycation

Protein glycation has a great deal to do with the damage that sugar causes in your body. But before you say "protein gly-what?" let me tell you that although it sounds technical, protein glycation is something you are likely very familiar with – it's something that probably happens every day in your very own kitchen.

Proteins and carbohydrates combine when brought together. This is especially the case in the presence of heat, or it can also happen through the use of enzymes. When a protein and a sugar combine, they form a new entity called a glycoprotein or glycated proteins. There are multiple ways in which proteins and carbohydrates can combine. Each has received the name of the scientist who discovered it: Amadori, Schiff base, and Maillard reactions. These reactions can proceed even further and create what are called Advanced Glycation End Products (AGEs).

Okay, this sounds complicated, but it really isn't. When you mix sugar and protein together, a chemical reaction takes place. This chemical reaction results in the creation of something new: a sugar-protein or a glycoprotein. In your kitchen, whenever you bake with sugar and protein, you produce glycated proteins. The most familiar glycated proteins form on the outside of the bread or cake you are cooking. For most of your life, you have known this as the *crust* or a browning reaction, but now you can properly call it a Maillard reaction, or the creation of glycated proteins.

While glycated proteins make for tasty bread or cake, they are actually disastrous when they are forming in your body. To form glycated proteins in your body all you have to do is provide the sugar for the reaction by drinking a soda or other sugar food, but the protein for the reaction comes from your body.

There are two kinds of proteins to which sugar can attach in your body. The first are free-flowing and found in the blood. These essential proteins do a lot for you; their main function is to transfer nutrients and other proteins throughout your body. The second kind of protein sugar can attach to are found on the cells of your blood vessels. When body blood vessel proteins become glycated serious destruction is occurring.[10] All of the toxic effects of sugar can be traced back to the damage it does to blood vessel proteins. High levels of sugar and subsequent protein glycation in diabetics have been proven to damage the blood vessels of the kidneys,[11] nerves,[12] and eyes.[13]

The big question, and the important question for people reading this book, is whether glycated proteins will affect a person *without* diabetes. If your blood sugar is in the normal range, are you still producing glycated proteins that cause damage? The answer to this question appears to be yes. People with normal blood sugar are still producing glycated proteins that cause damage to blood vessels.[14] The more sugary the meal, the more protein glycation takes place; conversely, eating lower on the glycemic index decreases the number of glycated proteins circulating in your body.[15]

This section wouldn't be finished without mentioning our friend fructose. Yes, as you may have guessed, fructose creates glycated proteins much more easily than does sucrose.[16] This confirms, once again, that you should avoid high fructose corn syrup like the plague.

From Small to Large

If high amounts of sugar cause destruction to the small blood vessels in the body, it makes sense that sugar may also be harmful to the larger blood vessels of the body. Scientists, in fact, are beginning to think this may be the case.

It is well known that diabetics are at a higher risk for atherosclerosis or hardening of the arteries. When the large blood vessels of the body are damaged by protein glycation, they tend to become clogged. Sugar attaches to the protein of the wall of the blood vessel and this damage is fixed by the body by using a cholesterol patch.[17] If enough of these patches are created, they eventually block the blood vessel entirely. In the heart these blockages are called coronary heart disease or clogged arteries and can lead to a heart attack. In the brain blockages may cause a stroke, while in the arms and legs, these blockages are called peripheral vascular disease.

Could sugar be the reason blood vessels begin to clog up in diabetics? I think there is a great deal more to be learned about atherosclerosis and the research is far from complete. However, since diabetics are two to four times more likely to develop heart disease and other blockages than non-diabetics, sugar is certainly a candidate for investigation as a contributing factor.

For the large blood vessels of the body, high blood sugar creates destruction through other means beyond protein glycation. High blood sugar also increases the presence of free radicals throughout the body, which in turn tends to increase bodily inflammation. When inflammatory chemicals are released into the blood stream, it causes a problem we talked about before: insulin resistance.[18] Insulin resistance leads to more sugar in the blood stream, which leads to free radical damage, which leads to more inflammation, which leads to more insulin resistance...so here we go again, spinning around in another end-less loop.

To make matters worse for the large blood vessels of the body, sugar in the blood stream also increases the factors that cause clotting and impairs the body's ability to break down clots.[19] This means that it is much easier to form clots in the blood stream and much more difficult to get rid of them. More clotting means a greater chance for a heart attack and other health problems.

And to think, all of this – insulin resistance, weight gain, heart disease, kidney disease, high blood pressure, and eye damage – began so innocently with a simple quest for something tasty to put into our mouths.

But Who's Counting?

Now, armed with the knowledge of what happens when sugar meets your body, which do you think causes more damage, cigarettes or sugar?

Roughly five million people worldwide die each year as a result of using tobacco.[20] That is a lot of people. But diabetes kills around three million people a year and this number continues to climb.[21] The United States and Canada have the *honor* of having a higher percentage of the population die from diabetes – eight percent. This is higher than some of the poorest countries in the world, where less than three percent of the population dies from diabetes. Apparently, being wealthy means you are more likely to get diabetes.

Comparing diabetes deaths with smoking deaths would make it appear that deaths due to sugar and cigarettes are roughly equal, especially in North America. But what happens if we include people who die due to other sugar-related deaths, such as obesity, heart disease, and stroke? Let's just look at one of those diseases: cardiovascular disease. Surely we cannot say that all the deaths due to cardiovascular disease are attributable to sugar, but a good portion of them are likely linked. Since heart disease and stroke account for one-third of all deaths, or around sixteen million people per year worldwide,[22] this makes the amount of destruction due to sugar much higher than that caused by cigarettes.

A Closer Look at Hypertension

For the most part, we have been discussing what happens when a high amount of sugar makes contact with your body, such as when someone has diabetes. There is no doubt that if you have diabetes, sugar has progressed from something tasty to something destructive. But what is the status for people who go to their doctors and are told that their blood sugar is normal? And what about those with pre-diabetes or metabolic syndrome? Remember, the risk of developing one of these sugar-related disorders over the course of the average person's lifetime is around fifty percent, perhaps higher. Can we blame heart, kidney, or eye diseases on sugar consumption in a supposedly normal person?

Take a look at hypertension and see what you think...

Hypertension, or high blood pressure, is a bit of a medical mystery. According to some estimates, over ninety percent of people who have hypertension have a kind of hypertension known as "essential hypertension" or "idiopathic hypertension," meaning that neither doctors nor scientists can find an underlying cause for the high blood pressure. It is estimated that one in five adults in the United States has hypertension (sixty million people worldwide).[23] That's a lot of people who have a disease for which medical science does not understand the cause.

Scientists are beginning to admit that sugar may have something to do with weight gain. If this is true, then sugar is at least partially responsible for high blood pressure. Your risk for high blood pressure increases with each pound you add over your ideal weight.

Let's also take a look back at what we know about high blood sugar in diabetics and what kind of damage sugar causes. We know that sugar is harmful to blood vessels in the kidneys and damage to the kidneys can result in high blood pressure. We also know that clogging of the arteries (atherosclerosis) is common in diabetics. When blood vessels are damaged with atherosclerosis, they become less flexible and more rigid; this also leads to increased blood pressure. Scientists can actually measure how elastic or flexible blood vessels are by a technical measurement called endothelial function and they note that diabetics have poor endothelial function. The good news is that when you gain control of blood sugar, endothelial function returns to normal.[24] In other words, controlling blood sugar means reversing much of the damage that has been done to blood vessels by high blood sugar.

Look at how sugar has the potential to cause hypertension through many mechanisms: weight gain, kidney damage, and blood vessel flexibility. Could sugar be the smoking gun we are looking for when we think about what is causing essential hypertension? Certainly in a diabetic, this is true.

The million dollar question is: Can this happen in people who are consuming *normal* levels of sugar and who show no sign of diabetes? Results from at least one study focused on this question and seem to suggest that fructose, at the very least, may contribute to hypertension through a variety of mechanisms.[25] Sugar seems to be, at least, a contributing factor in essential hypertension, if not the main causative factor.

The studies in this section mark the beginning of what I speculate will be many more studies that will arrive at the same conclusion. We can no longer ignore the role that sugar and sugar foods play in the development of many of the common diseases we encounter as we age. I admit it is a big leap to make, but what if we could avoid most cardiovascular, eye, kidney, nerve, and other diseases by avoiding sugar and foods that act like sugar? What if heart disease is not due to high cholesterol or inflammation, but instead is a result of ingesting sugar or foods that act like sugar? Only time and more studies will determine the truth. For now, you should consider that the foods you choose to put into your mouth can have a dramatic effect on your health and longevity.

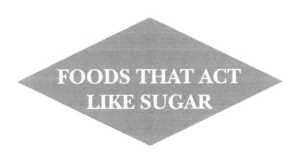

FOODS THAT ACT LIKE SUGAR

At this point, you may be thinking to yourself, "Okay, you convinced me, it may be hard to stop eating sugar, but I think I can do it." Before you decide to take that step, I have to explain something that I have mentioned throughout the book that will now make taking all the sugars out of your diet even harder! This is probably not what you wanted to hear at this point, but by reading this next section, you will gain valuable tools that will enable you to understand how to minimize the impact of sugars and foods that act like sugar on your body.

There it is again. Did you see it?

Throughout this book I have been using the phrase *sugars and foods that act like sugar*. Let me tell you exactly what I mean by *foods that act like sugar*. Remember that quote from the sugar industry earlier in the book? It went like this:

> *The available evidence from clinical studies demonstrates that dietary sucrose does not increase glycemia more than isocaloric amounts of starch. Thus, intake of sucrose and sucrose containing foods by people with diabetes does not need to be restricted because of concern about aggravating hyperglycemia.*

While I hate to admit that the sugar industry is correct, they are. Well, at least the first part of their statement is accurate. The second sentence when they talk of not needing to restrict sucrose or sucrose-containing foods is pure fuzzy thinking.

The sugar industry calls them "isocaloric starches" and I call them *foods that act like sugar in your body*, but they are the same thing. When you eat sugar, your blood sugar rises – you know this much already. But what happens when you eat these so-called isocaloric starches?

What you will discover is that comparing eating isocaloric starches to eating sugar is a bit like comparing drinking wine to drinking beer; they are not that different. The question that should be asked by all of us is not if isocaloric starches raise your blood sugar in the same way that table sugar does, but rather, should you be eating isocaloric starches at all?

Isocaloric Starches

The word iso means *the same* and caloric means the *amount of calories.* You learned about starches (carbohydrates) earlier and know that they are a simple carbohydrate. So what the sugar industry is saying when they use the term isocaloric starches is that when you compare the way sugar behaves to the behavior of the same amount of calories in a starch (carbohydrate), they will both increase blood sugar the same amount. This means that certain starches act exactly like sugar in your body.

Can this really be true?

Studies have been done, and, yes, these starches have the same effect on your blood sugar as table sugar. In fact, in the wacky world of the glycemic index, there are some isocaloric starches like white bread, or even rice cakes, which increase your blood sugar even more than eating straight table sugar! Think about what this means – certain starches act more like sugar than sugar. Now that you know about the destruction that sugar can cause in your blood stream, do you really think (like the sugar industry suggests) that you *do not* need to restrict sugar because there are starches that act the same as sugar? No, what you need to ask yourself is this: Should you be eating *any* foods that cause large spikes in your blood sugar? After all, 10,000 years ago, none of these foods were a part of our diet.

There are two approaches to dealing with foods that can rapidly increase your blood sugar. The first is to simply avoid them, and the second is to learn how to keep your blood sugar low even if you are eating them. How do you keep your blood sugar low while still eating these foods? For answers, we turn to the concept of the glycemic index.

Enter the Glycemic Index

For years scientists and doctors made assumptions about which carbohydrates would increase blood sugar, mostly based on carbohydrate content inside the food. This, it turns out, is not a very accurate way to measure what is going on inside the body when we eat these foods. These assumptions went unchallenged for years until it occurred to a researcher to actually test how foods act inside the body and to monitor what these foods do to blood sugar levels.

Out of this research was born the glycemic index.

The glycemic index is a measure of how much an individual food increases blood sugar. It works like this: First a scientist measures a volunteer's blood sugar. The volunteer eats a single food and after a certain amount of time (usually an hour later), the volunteer's blood sugar level is again measured. Through exhaustive research of this kind, scientists have been able to determine how different foods affect our blood sugar levels.

What we have discovered using the glycemic index has been amazing. Here are some typical glycemic index values for common carbohydrates:

Carbohydrate	Glycemic Index
Glucose	100
Instant Mashed Potatoes	97
White Rice	98
Baguette	95
Baked Potato	94
Corn Flakes	80
Sucrose	70

Here is what you need to know to read the glycemic index: Any food that measures over 70 is considered a high-glycemic food and low-glycemic foods measure below 55 on the scale. High glycemic index foods increase blood sugar dramatically, while low glycemic foods don't affect blood sugar much. What you have to remember is what, exactly, the glycemic index measuring. When the glycemic index is measuring blood sugar levels, it is measuring the amount of *glucose* in the blood, not other sugars, such as fructose. The importance of this distinction will become obvious later in the book.

As you can see from the above chart, many foods increase blood sugar at least as much as, if not more than, eating pure sucrose (table sugar). Armed with this information from the glycemic index, you can now understand what the sugar industry means when it says that isocaloric starches act similarly to the way sugar does in the body. Isocaloric starches like potatoes, corn flakes, rice, and others *look* just like sugar to your body. In fact, when you eat these isocaloric starchy foods, your blood sugar level is going to rise just as if you had eaten several spoonfuls of white sugar.

You Are What You Eat

Now let's briefly take on the more important question: Should you even be eating isocaloric starches? As you now know, sugar, grains, and starchy vegetables are a relatively new addition to the human diet. While we have seen a steady increase in the amount of grains and sugars in our diets over the last few thousands years, the real jump in the number of sugars and foods that act like sugar in our diets has taken place only during the last one or two hundred years.

Anthropologists actually have a lot to say about if we should be eating sugars and foods that act like sugar. When they studied what happened when hunter-gatherer peoples changed from their traditional diet to growing grains (around 10,000 years ago), anthropologists discovered that the peoples who changed to agriculture actually lost height.[1] Not only that, but the hunters-turned-farmers demonstrated a decrease in the relative level of their health that was measurable in their bones. Osteoporosis and tooth decay were much more common in farmers than in their cousins who continued to hunt and gather.

A pioneering dentist by the name of Weston Price traveled the globe in the 1930s studying people who were making the transition from traditional hunter-gatherer diets to more Western diets (full of sugars foods). He discovered relatives, such as brothers, where one had changed to a Western diet and the other had continued with a traditional diet. When he compared the two, he was astounded. The siblings who were eating the Western diets had experienced changes to their bodies that were noticeable to Dr. Price. As a dentist, he focused much of his study on teeth and noticed that Western diets *produced* people whose mouths were much narrower, more crowded, and, of course, more cavity-ridden than those who ate traditional diets. However, there were other noticeable changes to the health and facial structures of those who had shifted to a Western diet.

If grains and starches are such optimal foods for us to eat, if they make up the bulk of what we are supposed to put into our mouths according to governmental agencies, scientists, doctors and the food pyramid, it is logical that we should see people become healthier when they choose a grain-based diet. This is simply not the case. Think back to your garden. If you provide plants with the right nutrients, they grow bigger and are less prone to disease. Human beings are no different.

Ultimately, only you can decide if grains and sugars are right for you and your health. As I mentioned before, you have a choice between completely eliminating them from your diet, or learning how to keep your blood sugar level low even when you are eating them. To understand how to make the second option work, we need to, once again, turn to the glycemic index.

A Closer Look at the Glycemic Index

Let's take a look at a selection of typical foods and see how they rate on the glycemic index:

The Glycemic Index of Select Foods

	SUGARS	GRAINS	GRAIN FOODS	FRUITS	VEGETABLES	BEANS	NUTS	
HIGH GLYCEMIC FOODS	Sucrose	White Rice						110
	Glucose Fruit Roll up		Pancakes	Dates				100
	Honey	Popcorn	Baguette Corn Flakes Rice Cracker		Parsnips Instant Potato Baked Potato Boiled Carrots			90
			Special K Pretzels					80
	Jelly Beans		Grape Nuts Donuts Wonder Bread Pop Tarts	Watermelon Banana	Sweet Potato Boiled Potato	Broad Beans Kidney Beans		70
MEDIUM	Coca Cola	Brown Rice Quick Oats		Pineapple Raisins Cherries				60
		Sweet Corn Long Rice	Bran Muffin Oatmeal Cookie	Black Grapes Peach Orange Juice				55
LOW GLYCEMIC FOODS			Fettucine Macaroni Spaghetti	Kiwi Apple Bartlett Pear Strawberries	Yam	Pinto Beans Chickpeas Baked Beans		40
		Pearl Barley	Meat Ravioli	Dried Apple		Butter Beans Blackeyed peas		30
	Xylitol			Cherries		Lima Beans Black Beans Lentils	Peanuts Cashews	20
	Fructose							10

There are a few things you want to notice about this chart. Notice first that most sugars and grains appear at the top of the chart and are considered high-glycemic foods. The grains that appear at the bottom of the chart are those containing a lot of fiber such as barley and are often eaten in whole-form (the way most people eat rice). Pastas also tend to be lower on the glycemic index because they tend to be a bit harder for your digestive system to break down, releasing sugars slowly into the blood stream. This is a good thing. You should also notice that there are high, medium, and low-glycemic fruits and that beans and nuts are generally low on the glycemic index.

Have you also noticed that there are numerous foods that are missing from this chart? Scientists measure only foods that will increase blood sugar, so you won't find any foods that don't increase blood sugar on this chart. These foods are what I would call *below the glycemic index* foods and they are foods that you can eat without worrying about how they will affect your blood sugar. It is not difficult to guess which foods these are; they are the same foods you found in the fields 10,000 years ago. These foods include many vegetables such as broccoli, onions, cabbage, garlic, Brussels sprouts, and greens of all kinds. They also include all of the proteins that come from animals, including meats, whey, and eggs. Eating foods from below the glycemic index is one of the healthiest ways that you can eat.

I should stop right here and tell you that I am not advocating a high protein diet, such as the Atkins diet. I will have a lot more to say about just how to structure a diet plan that will work for you later in the book.

What is Wrong with the Glycemic Index?

You should also know that the glycemic index is not perfect. The way I presented it above makes it appear as though the glycemic index value for a certain food is clear and straightforward. This is not entirely the case. If you look up what the glycemic index for a certain food is, you will find that it can vary depending on where you find the information. In some charts you may find oranges listed as a high glycemic index food while in another chart you may find them listed as a low glycemic index food. The reasons for this are many, and are the result of different scientific teams testing similar foods.

The two most likely reasons scientists don't get consistent results when they test for glycemic index are that foods vary as do our responses to them.

Anyone who has ever farmed, or been a gardener, will know that soil is highly variable. Identical plants planted a few feet apart can grow differently and produce different food quality. Additionally, an orange picked early in the season, may have less sugar content than one picked later. An orange grown in Florida that was tested for the glycemic index may be completely different than one grown in Spain.

People are also variable; we each may react differently to the same food. If you and I were, for example, to eat oranges, my blood sugar may rise higher than yours, but when we ate carrots, yours may become higher than mine.

The glycemic index is also a very poor predictor for what happens when someone eats more than one food at the same time. Remember that when they test for glycemic index, only one food for each test is used. What happens when you eat a meal of mixed foods? You would think that if you ate a high-glycemic index food and mixed it with a low-glycemic food that your blood sugar would be somewhere in the middle. This is often not the case.

While the glycemic index is not perfect, this doesn't mean it should be dismissed entirely. Scientists are working on perfecting the glycemic index by adding a calculation to the formula that takes into account the amount of food being eaten. This new measurement is called glycemic load and this may prove to be more helpful, but needs further study to determine just how well it works for people trying to keep their blood sugar low.

The best way to use the glycemic index is to think of it more as a guideline than a rule book. The glycemic index suggests that sugars, grains, and certain starchy vegetable and fruits will cause your blood sugar to spike more than if you are eating, say, a steak. That is good information to have when you sit down to your dinner table. If you hope to live a long and healthy life, you should try to eat as many foods as possible that are below or off the glycemic index. Later in the book, using the glycemic index as a guide, I will steer you in the direction of eating to keep your blood sugar low.

Now, though, is a good time to stop and take a look at the other kinds of sweeteners that have made their way into our diets.

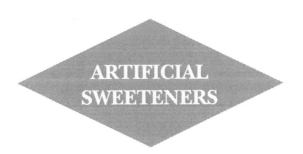

ARTIFICIAL SWEETENERS

As if the last chapter wasn't painful enough! First I told you that you would have to remove the white death, table sugar, from your life. Then I told you that you shouldn't stop there, that you have to remove or limit foods that act like sugar in your body. Now I'm about to make your journey to remove and keep sugars out of your diet even more difficult.

You probably know what I'm going to say about artificial sweeteners, don't you? What you may not expect is that I would actually recommend that you eat real sugar before you ever touch another food with an artificial sweetener in it again. After all that you have learned about how harmful sugars and foods that act like sugar are, you may be surprised by that suggestion, but that is how harmful I think these artificial sweeteners really are.

Artificial sweeteners have become the darlings of doctors and scientists. From the perspective of medical science, artificial sweeteners seem like the perfect substitute for sugar: All the sweet taste and no calories. In fact, soda companies are calculating that very soon they will be producing more soda with artificial sweeteners than those with regular sugars. Artificial sweeteners make it seem as if you can really have your cake and eat it too, but as my grandmother used to warn me, *nothing in the world is free.* While on the surface artificial sweeteners appear to have all the benefits and none of the down sides of sugar, the truth is that they are not all the advertising has led you to believe. There is a high price you body pays for using them.

When you think about it, all sweeteners you encounter are artificial. I've said this enough throughout this book, but I'll say it again: Concentrated sugars simply don't exist in nature (with the exception of honey). While we can't find high fructose corn syrup or table sugar in nature, the molecules that make them up (glucose, fructose) are found throughout nature. It would be truly remarkable, though, to find bees that could manufacture something like Splenda, Equal, or NutraSweet. These molecules are alien to both our planet and your body.

My intention with this chapter is not to cover the whole topic of artificial sweeteners, but to simply make you aware of some of the controversy surrounding these non-foods. Other books do an excellent job of covering this subject in more detail. *Aspartame: Is it Safe?* by H.J. Roberts is a well-researched classic on the subject and the more recent *Sweet Deception* by Mercola and Pearsall is another great read, covering many artificial sweeteners and the health issues surrounding them.

The History of Artificial Sweeteners

The history of artificial sweeteners is a fascinating one. Almost every one of these fake sugars was discovered by accident. The story usually goes like this: A chemist working on another project accidentally tastes the chemical they are working on and, instead of dying, discovered a new artificial sweetener.

Saccharin was the first of these accidents. Saccharin was dis-covered in 1879 when a John Hopkins researcher spilled an experimental chemical on his finger and accidentally touched his mouth; he was surprised by the sweetness. Luckily for him, saccharin was not immediately harmful. Saccharin lived in ob-scurity for many years until cane sugar became scarce and was rationed during World Wars I and II. The shortage of real sug-ar led to a search for an alternative and saccharin made its way into everyday products and even into troop rations.

Saccharin is about three hundred times sweeter than table sugar, but has a bad metallic aftertaste. Unlike many artificial sweeteners, it can be heated and mixed into cooked foods. Saccharin became increasingly popular until the 1960s when it was found to cause bladder cancer in lab rats. Although it was never banned in the United States, other countries have banned its use. Public outcry to the use of saccharin and the poor aftertaste has placed saccharin on the back shelf. In re-cent years, manufacturers have begun to use it again by blend-ing it with other sweeteners to mask the aftertaste.

Aspartame was discovered in 1965 through another accidental tasting by James Schlatter, and was given approval by the United States Food and Drug Administration (FDA) in 1981. Acesul-fame potassium, also known as Acesulfame K or Ace K, was discovered by a German chemical company and was approved for use by the FDA in 1992. Sucralose, or Splenda, is the latest of the chemical sweeteners to be discovered and approved for use by the FDA in foods and beverages in 1998.

In the Body

What happens when you eat these non-foods is largely un-known. Studies in lab animals have been done, but once the sweetener is approved, ongoing toxicity research is rare. There is an ongoing experiment with artificial sweeteners, though, and it happens every day as millions of people reach for their diet sodas. The results of this "experiment" add to our already poor health and obesity epidemic.

Saccharin

Saccharin passes directly through the human digestive system without being digested, or at least this is what the chemical companies who manufacture it claim. Chemical companies defend saccharin by saying that it was shown to cause bladder cancer in rats only by giving them very large doses; this is true. But considering all the foods that artificial sweeteners appear in today, it would not be too hard to get a large dose of saccharin. Scientific studies, with rats and saccharin, also tend to be short (a few weeks or months), and say nothing about the long term effects of a chemical like saccharin, which is likely where the danger lies. One has to wonder, though, how bladder cancer happens in rats when saccharin supposedly passes through their bodies without being digested.

Aspartame

Aspartame (also known as Nutrasweet or Equal) is comprised of a chemical molecule that breaks down into aspartate, phenylalanine, and methanol when digested. In case you were wondering, the first two breakdown products (aspartate and phenylalanine) are amino acids or proteins. The last, methanol, is an alcohol and is poisonous to human beings. Methanol can cause liver, brain, and eye damage when taken in large amounts. Manufacturers know that methanol is toxic, but claim there is so little in Aspartame that it shouldn't affect humans. This might make sense except that manufacturers are required to warn people with a rare genetic disorder called phenylketonuria that they should avoid aspartame use. People with phenylketonuria are sensitive to phenylalanine (one of the amino acid breakdown product) and must not use aspartame even though there is only a small amount in the product.

Even if aspartame contains a small amount of a toxic substance, methanol, you have to wonder what happens when you consume it over a long period of time. Many health-oriented doctors report that their patients who suffer from a wide variety of common conditions, such as headache, fatigue, digestive complaints, and so on, often improve by simply removing all artificial sweeteners from their diet.

Aspartame was originally shown to cause brain cancer in rats. This finding caused the FDA to hold back approval for a while, but eventually they gave it the go ahead. New research of the link between aspartame consumption, cancer, and other diseases is ongoing. The most interesting study used rats and small doses of aspartame over time, the relative equivalent of what would be considered a typical, real-life exposure to the chemical. This study reported an increase in the amount of cancers in rats;[1] another long term study had similar findings.[2]

H.J. Roberts, MD, who coined the term *aspartame disease*, reports that aspartame has been linked to headache, dizziness, mood shifts, nausea and vomiting, abdominal pain and cramps, joint pain, vision changes, slurred speech, diarrhea, seizures, memory loss, numbness and cramping in arms and legs, and fatigue. Aspartame is linked to diseases including fibromyalgia, tinnitus (ringing in the ear), depression, anxiety attacks, multiple sclerosis, systemic lupus, and various cancers.

In 1995, FDA Epidemiology Branch Chief Thomas Wilcox stated that aspartame complaints represented seventy-five percent of all reports of adverse reactions to substances in the food supply between 1981 and 1995.[3] That is a lot of complaints about a single food additive; still, aspartame remains on our shelves.

Sucralose

Sucralose (Splenda) is also supposedly not absorbed by the body. Sucralose is a molecule that belongs to a group of molecules known as organochlorides. As a group, organochlorides are some of the most toxic substances on earth. Even small amounts of certain organochlorides can be extremely toxic. While this *guilt by association* doesn't prove the harmfulness of sucralose, it should cause scientists and consumers to take a very close look at this molecule before ingesting it. The FDA considers sucralose to be safe based on over one hundred scientific studies. Not everyone is convinced.

In a strange twist of fate, it is the sugar industry that has become one of the strongest opponents to Splenda. The sugar industry launched a site called the Truth about Splenda, citing safety and other concerns. Here is what the sugar industry has to say about Splenda:

Fiction: Splenda is safe to eat, even for children.

Fact: There are no conclusive tests that support this statement. Again, there have been no long-term human studies conducted to determine the potential health effects of Splenda on humans, including children. Until long-term human studies are conducted, no one will know for sure whether Splenda is really safe or unsafe for humans to eat.

And again:

Fiction: Splenda has been thoroughly tested.

Fact: There has not been a single long-term human study to determine the potential health effects of Splenda on people. The FDA relied on a few short-term tests when it reviewed the safety of Splenda for human consumption. Worse, these human tests were all conducted by the manufacturer of Splenda, hardly an unbiased source. The vast majority of tests reviewed by the FDA to determine whether Splenda was safe for human consumption were conducted on animals, including rats and rabbits.

I find myself in the unlikely position of actually agreeing with the sugar industry. The reports of illnesses associated with sucralose are increasing. One small study has already suggested that sucralose may be responsible for the increase in the number of migraine headache patients.[4]

Acesulfame K

Acesulfame K stimulates the secretion of insulin; this can lead to low blood sugar.

Studies indicate Acesulfame K can cause breast, thymus, and lung tumors. This sweetener has been shown to cause chronic respiratory disease and leukemia in lab animals. The Center for Science in the Public Interest has petitioned the FDA to remove Acesulfame K from the market because of *significant doubt* about the safety of the molecule.

Lack of Study

One of the most serious problems with artificial sweeteners and, really, any food additive that the FDA approves, is that many of the scientific tests are conducted on animals over the short term. As much as researchers may try, laboratory tests don't mimic real life when human beings are consuming these artificial chemicals on a daily basis. It may very well be okay for you to use artificial sweeteners once or twice a month, but ingesting them daily is likely where the potential for harm occurs.

Another point to consider is that the chemicals that make up these sweeteners are new to the world. This is no small point. Human beings have co-evolved along with their food for millions of years. It is estimated that over one thousand new chemicals are introduced into our foods every year. Your body can be confused by these strange chemicals and must find ways to cope with them. This places a large burden on the body's detoxification systems, such as the liver and kidney. The risks associated with using artificial sweeteners are far greater than their so-called benefits.

Cravings Do Not Go Away

Here is the crux of the problem with artificial sweeteners: They don't do what you want them to do. You reach for artificial sweeteners because you think choosing them will help to reduce the amount of calories you are consuming. This simply doesn't happen. Some studies show that when you are drinking artificially sweetened drinks, the total amount of calories you eat actually increases.[5]

Why do you eat more if you are drinking artificially sweetened drinks? The answer is probably that you are tricking your body.

Whenever you put something sweet into your mouth, you set off a whole series of processes, including the release of hormones, all cued to digest the food you eat. When no calories actually arrive, your body becomes confused.

Many artificial sweeteners cause insulin levels to rise in your blood. This creates problems when all you are doing is drinking a soda with no other foods. Up goes insulin and this (remember?) means that any sugar in your blood will move into cells, reducing your blood sugar. The end result of eating artificial sweeteners, especially when it is a soda, is lowered blood sugar. When you have low blood sugar, you are going to be hungry and crave more food. And, more to the point of the issues covered in this book, as long as you are putting a sweet taste into your mouth, you are continuing your addiction to sweetness. If you go on a program where you are reducing or eliminating sugars in your life, your taste buds will reset to a lower sweet taste. You will be surprised how sweet apples, peaches, berries, and other fruits taste after you have weaned yourself off the super-sweet taste of sugars and artificial sweeteners.

Do yourself a favor and don't add to the burden your body already has: remove all artificial sweeteners from your life.

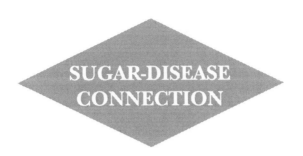

SUGAR-DISEASE CONNECTION

By the time you get to this chapter in the book, you may be tired of scientific studies and ready to learn what you can do to eliminate sugars from your life. Or, if you are going to still eat sugar foods, you probably want to learn how to reduce the impact that they have on your health. If this is what you're looking for now, feel free to skip over this chapter. If you have the patience to carry on, though, this chapter will review the connection between sugar and many common diseases in more detail. The evidence connecting sugar and foods that act like sugar with disease is growing, but somehow the medical communities continue to ignore the clinical studies that show a connection between sugar and disease. Since you aren't going to read it anywhere else, this chapter will show you what the scientific community is saying about the sugar-disease connection.

Let's Visit the So-Called Experts

The people who should be telling you that sugar and foods that act like sugar cause disease are not doing their job. Organizations, such as the American Diabetes Association, The World Health Organization, and others – whose job it is to set policy on health topics – are strangely silent on the subject of sugar and how it affects your health. These associations should be providing guidelines for living a longer and healthier life, but are they really doing this?

Let's stop by the websites of a few of these associations to see what they have to say about sugar in your diet. Can you guess which website provided this advice?

> *For many years, people with diabetes were told to avoid sugar at all costs. It was thought that sugar would pass into the bloodstream faster and easier and would cause blood glucose levels to rise too quickly. More recent research has shown that all carbohydrates affect blood glucose levels the same way. A potato and a brownie, if they have the same number of carbohydrates, have about the same affect on blood glucose levels....There is no reason, however, for your child to avoid all sugary foods. In the context of a healthy diet, an occasional candy bar or bowl of ice cream should cause no problems for her diabetes control. You do need to plan for the inclusion of sweets in her diet to ensure that she has enough insulin in her system to handle the carbohydrates in the sweets.*[1]

This quote is from the American Diabetes Association is key to the problems with current medical thinking. The American Diabetes Association has learned, as you have, that the glycemic index of a brownie is similar to the glycemic index of a potato. But instead of saying that you should stay away from both of these foods, they have concluded that both are okay to eat. Well, they say, it is okay to eat them as long as your diabetic child is taking enough insulin. This is sheer craziness! The number of people with diabetes is growing every day and yet, they think it is just fine for diabetics to eat sugars as long as they are taking enough artificial insulin. Even the American Diabetes Association's respected scientific journal, *Diabetes Care*, in a review of sugar has this to say:

Data currently available indicate that high sucrose consumption does not contribute significantly to the prevalence of cardiovascular disease, diabetes mellitus, obesity, or micronutrient deficiency. It may contribute, however, to dental caries formation by cariogenic bacteria.[2]

Sugar causes no harm, except for hurting your teeth; you will hear this lunacy over and over again. Another association, the American Dietetic Association – the association that registers dietitians – has this to say about sugar:

Although the new Dietary Guidelines for Americans don't set a specific cap on sugar, if you consume foods in the proportions recommended for your particular calorie level, it's tough to take in too much sugar. Nevertheless, it's a good idea to try to limit portions, especially when you consume sugary foods such as candy, nondiet soda, juices that aren't 100% fruit juice, cakes, cookies, jams and jellies, to name a few.

The Dietary Reference Intake Reports of the National Academy of Sciences Food and Nutrition boards currently suggests that not more than 25% of your total calories should come from added sugars.[3]

The American Dietetic Association first says that it is tough to "take in too much sugar," and then cites the dietary recommendations from the National Academy of Sciences, which suggests that no more than twenty-five percent of your total calories should come from added sugars. Read that again: 25 percent of your total calories from *added* sugars. So it looks as though one quarter (how can this be possible?) of your diet can be sucrose or high fructose corn syrup with, supposedly, no ill effects on your health. And, no mention of foods that act like sugar from the American Dietetic Association – apparently you can eat as many of these as you like.

The World Health Organization (WHO) is also in agreement with this sugar advice. According to the WHO, there is no direct link between consumption of sugars and heart disease, diabetes, and other chronic diseases. The WHO at least acknowledges that sugar does have calories, and if you eat too many calories you are bound to gain weight, and this weight gain raises your risk for diabetes and heart disease.[4]

I could go on and on; each group or association that is supposed to help you make decisions about your health is constantly giving incorrect advice. If their advice was so great, wouldn't we see a decrease in the number of people with diabetes and obesity? Wouldn't people be healthier? Despite what the above associations may be saying, there is research to support that sugar does have an impact on our health. Let's take a look.

Obesity

In general, the medical community does not consider sugar to be harmful to your health. They may be, however, starting to change their minds about the connection between sugar and weight gain. In truth, they have to change their minds; the number of scientific studies that connect sugar and foods that act like sugar with weight gain is growing almost as fast as the epidemic of obesity.

Obesity is out of control. The medical costs associated with obese patients in the United States top 75 billion dollars a year and continue to climb. Over half of all of these costs are paid for through government programs, such as Medicare and Medicaid. This places an enormous burden on all tax payers; other countries are facing similar expenses. Deaths associated with obesity are expected to soon top those due to cancer or heart disease. Obesity may become the number one cause of death in developed countries.[5]

Direct or Indirect?

The medical community admits that sugar may cause weight gain, but only because sugar is part of all the calories that you consume every day. To understand exactly what they are saying, you first have to understand the concept of direct and indirect causes. This is a pretty straight forward concept, but it has wide-reaching implications.

Direct causes are those causes that can be blamed directly on something. Indirect causes are those causes that may have an influence, but are not directly to blame. For instance, if sugar makes you fat, you could say that sugar is a direct cause of obesity. The more sugar you eat, the fatter you are going to become.

While scientific studies are now illustrating that sugar does have a *direct* effect on weight gain, the medical communities are more likely to admit that sugar has an *indirect* effect on weight gain.

The claim that sugar has an indirect effect on weight gain goes something like this: Sugar contains calories and calories cause weight gain so the more calories that someone eats, the more they are likely to gain weight. Did you get that? It is a bit subtle, but an important point. Sugar, in their view, may contribute to weight gain, but only because – like any other food you eat – it contains calories. As we proceed through this section, you will learn that sugar does cause weight gain because it contains calories, but it also causes weight gain just *because it is sugar!* There is something about sugar that leads to weight gain, more than the fact that it just contains calories.

I bring up this discussion of direct and indirect because as we consider the rest of the diseases in which sugar may play a role, you need to know that obesity has a huge *indirect* effect on other diseases. If you are obese, your risk for many other diseases skyrockets.

According to the Centers for Disease Control, obesity increases the risk for the following diseases:

- Coronary heart disease
- Dyslipidemia (high total cholesterol or triglycerides)
- Gallbladder disease
- Hypertension (high blood pressure)
- Osteoarthritis (the break down of cartilage and bone within a joint)
- Sleep apnea and respiratory problems
- Some cancers (lining of the uterus, breast, and colon)
- Stroke
- Type 2 diabetes

Obesity does not cause all of these diseases, but the risk for getting them greatly increases if you are overweight. While the studies below illustrate that sugar has a direct effect on weight gain (and other diseases), it is useful to remember the indirect effects of obesity. If you conclude that sugar is responsible for weight gain, you have to admit that sugar is at least partly responsible for heart disease, diabetes, stroke, and even cancer.

Sugar Causes Obesity

Yes, sugar does contribute to weight gain because it contains calories, but sugar also causes weight gain simply because it is sugar.

Sugar, unlike other foods, is easily converted into fat in your body and you are compelled to keep putting it in your mouth because it is addictive. While the medical community is reluctant to admit that sugar directly causes weight gain, you already know (from earlier chapters) how this works: If your blood sugar rises after a meal, your body somehow has to deal with the increase in blood sugar. One of the ways your body deals with excess sugar is to store that energy as fat. Remember, fructose makes this conversion from blood sugar to body fat especially easily.[6]

Anyone who has ever tried a high protein diet, such as Atkins or South Beach, knows that avoiding carbohydrates and sugars lead to weight loss. Calories don't really matter as much as you have been led to believe. Eating the identical amount of calories from a sugar and a protein leads to different results in your body. Sugar behaves differently in your body because it is easily absorbed and just as easily turned into fat. But sugar doesn't stop with just being easily turned into fat; it is as addictive as cigarettes, alcohol, and opioids.

When the food that causes you to gain weight is also the same food that you are addicted to, you have a recipe (pun intended) for weight gain. Every time you try to go on a diet, you will come face-to-face with your addiction and begin to crave the very thing that keeps adding pounds.

High Glycemic Foods

If you were to create a diet based on what the conventional wisdom is about sugars and carbohydrates, you would follow the food pyramid – or some other advice – and create a diet that is heavily based on grains, fruits, and vegetables. This kind of diet, however, doesn't take into account that many of these foods act identically to sugar, or as one research study put it:

> *There is consensus that carbohydrate foods, in the form of fruit, vegetables and whole-grain products, are beneficial to health. However, there are strong indications that highly processed, fibre-depleted, and consequently rapidly digestible, energy-dense carbohydrate food products can lead to over-consumption and obesity-related diseases.*[7]

Carbohydrates are unique among foods that we eat. Most people can sit down and eat a large amount of carbohydrates, but this isn't true of other foods. We have already discussed how common it is to binge on carbohydrates. A large plate of spaghetti, a bag of potato chips, a container of ice cream; all these carbohydrates are addictive. You just don't seem to fill up as much as you do when eating the same amount of steak, broccoli, or even apples. The sheer volume of carbohydrates you can eat is enormous because they are addictive.

What the Studies Show

Scientists have taken on the study of sugar and foods that act like sugar and how they affect appetite, amount of calories consumed, and weight gain. The bulk of these studies focus on what happens when people eat high glycemic index foods. Here is what they found:

In a rat study, when sugar was available, the rats consumed over thirty percent more calories than they did when sugar was not available.[8]

-Psychological Reports, 2002

In a long-term study of normal weight and obese children between the ages of nine and twelve, researchers found that a low glycemic index breakfast, and even low glycemic index breakfast with ten percent sugar, was better at reducing appetite throughout the day than a typical high-sugar breakfast.[9]

- Pediatrics, 2003

While this might seem obvious, researchers in this study discovered that small meals produce a small rise in insulin and other hormones, while large meals produce large amounts of insulin and other hormones. This is true even when the meals are *high glycemic index* meals.[10]

-Nutrition Journal, 2006

The following are reviews. Remember that reviews hold more weight than individual studies because researchers gather information from many studies to complete their review.

A review of forty-five studies showed that eating foods that are lower on the glycemic index kept both fasting blood glucose and glycated proteins lower (remember that glycated proteins are one of the main ways in which sugar can cause damage in your body). Adding fiber to the diet helped keep blood sugar levels low. Most of the studies illustrated that eating low-glycemic foods increases insulin sensitivity, reduces triglycerides, and lowers body weight.[11]

-American Journal of Clinical Nutrition, 2008

In another review, researchers point out that eating low-glycemic food reduces the risk for diabetes and coronary heart disease, and improves the likelihood of healthy levels of high-density lipoprotein (HDL) cholesterol, triglycerides, C-reactive protein, and glycated proteins in the body.[12]

-*The Proceedings of the Nutrition Society, 2005*

One of the most respected reviews in medicine is called a Cochrane Review. When a topic is examined in a Cochrane review, you can be assured that their statements are backed up by a large amount of research. Here is what the Cochrane Review has to say about eating low-glycemic meals and how doing so affects our health:

"Body mass, total fat mass, body mass index, total cholesterol and LDL-cholesterol all decreased significantly more in the Low Glycemic Index group. In studies comparing Low Glycemic Index diets to conventional restricted energy low-fat diets, participants fared as well or better on the Low Glycemic Index diet, even though they could eat as much as desired. Lowering the glycemic load of the diet appears to be an effective method of promoting weight loss and improving lipid profiles and can be simply incorporated into a person's lifestyle."[13]

-*Cochrane Database of Systematic Reviews, 2007*

So what did we learn from these studies?

- The study on children who eat high sugar breakfasts illustrates what I call "the sugar magnet" – once you eat sugar, you simply want more. A high glycemic index meal induces a series of hormonal changes that lead to more cravings throughout the day.
- The research on small meals resulting in small insulin responses, regardless if the meal is a high glycemic, il-

lustrates the importance of eating small meals (versus large ones) throughout the day to keep insulin levels low.

- Increasing fiber helps to keep blood sugar down.
- A low glycemic index diet is just as effective as a low-fat and low-calorie diet for losing weight, even when you can eat as much as you want of low glycemic foods.
- All of these studies illustrate that by eating meals considered to be low glycemic, you can improve many aspects of your health, including weight loss.

So there you have it: Sugar has both a direct and indirect effect on weight gain. Why the medical community isn't screaming this message is difficult to understand. When reviewing the rest of the diseases that may be caused by sugar, keep in mind the indirect relationship between increased weight and disease.

Diabetes

We have already reviewed the steps in the development of diabetes in an earlier chapter. When sugar hits your blood stream in large amounts, your body has to somehow adjust. The choices that your body makes when your blood sugar is high aren't necessarily the best ones for you in the long run, but your body is making the best of a bad situation. When we constantly eat sugar foods, we are creating a situation whereby insulin insensitivity, metabolic syndrome, and diabetes are much more likely to happen.

So you would think I could show you a mountain of research that supports the connection between diabetes and sugar intake, but I can't. The funny thing about connecting diabetes to sugar intake is that it is so obvious: Wouldn't a poor sugar-control disease be caused by eating too much sugar? Apparently this has not occurred to many researchers.

All along, the research challenge has been the difficulty of finding an adequate control group – that is, a group that is not eating sugars or foods that act like sugar – for comparison. Where on earth can scientists find people who are not eating a large amount of grains or sugars? Not too many places.

There is a general agreement in the scientific community that when people who live in more rural areas of the world move to an area that is more urban, they experience an increase in obesity, diabetes and other diseases.[14] Scientists blame this increase on *lifestyle factors,* but are at a loss to explain exactly which lifestyle factor is causing diabetes and weight gain to surface. People who live in more rural areas tend to eat more traditional diets; when they move to the city, they switch to more processed foods and fewer fruits and vegetables.

When scientists discovered the glycemic index, they found the key to the reason why we have seen a spike in the number of people with diabetes. The glycemic index told them that there are foods that we eat every day that act identical to sugar. When they discovered this fact, they had two choices. The first was to conclude that since sugar acts similarly to other foods, both are okay to eat. They could have also concluded that since sugar acts identically to other foods, we shouldn't be eating either of them. These scientists ignored the fact that there have been dramatic changes to our diets at various stages in human history and they chose option number one: Both sugar and foods that act like sugar are okay to eat. Don't you make that same mistake.

As I mentioned above, medical researchers admit that sugar has indirect effects on diabetes. Sugar *may* lead to weight gain and the more overweight you are, the higher the risk of diabetes.[15] But this is not a very strong statement considering all that we have learned in these last several chapters.

We have discussed diabetes throughout this book, but you should remember that your risk of getting diabetes is around thirty percent. This means that one-third of the people who are reading this book will get diabetes sometime in their lives. For a large amount of people, this disease goes unnoticed. It is estimated that there are over six million people with diabetes in the United States who don't even know they have the disease.[16] This is a large number of people who are walking around with a damaging disease of which they aren't aware.

While you have read about many of the problems associated with diabetes throughout this book (higher risk for heart disease, stroke, kidney disease, blindness, nerve problems, and other diseases), it is also important to know that diabetes will shorten your lifespan. An individual diagnosed with diabetes at forty years of age will typically lose nearly twelve years (for men) and about fourteen years (for women) from their life expectancy.[17]

When the medical community talks about what causes diabetes, they mostly speak in terms of risk factors. Being overweight causes diabetes, a sedentary lifestyle causes diabetes; some even go as far as saying insulin insensitivity is what causes diabetes. But almost no one is talking about the real cause of insulin insensitivity and diabetes: sugar and foods that act like sugar.

As recently as January, 2008, medical literature is saying:

> *Interest in the glycemic impact of diet on health and well-being is growing among health care professionals and consumers. Diets with high glycemic impact [sugars and foods that act like sugar]*

have been postulated to increase risk of obesity, insulin resistance, diabetes, and cardiovascular disease...Yet, a scientific debate exists about whether a relation between the glycemic response to diet and health truly exists...lower Glycemic Index and Glycemic Load diets are beneficial for health in persons with impaired glucose metabolism [people with diabetes and metabolic syndrome], but it is as yet unclear what they mean for healthy persons.[18]

Surprisingly, there is still a scientific debate on the role of sugar in diabetes. Another review, discussing how to prevent type 2 diabetes, had this to say:

Based on the strength of available evidence regarding diet and lifestyle in the prevention of type 2 diabetes, it is recommended that a normal weight status in the lower Body Mass Index (BMI) range (BMI 21-23) and regular physical activity be maintained throughout adulthood; abdominal obesity be prevented; and saturated fat intake be less than 7% of the total energy intake.[19]

They just aren't connecting the dots or thinking the next thought. In order to prevent diabetes, they say, you need to exercise and keep your body weight normal. But what about sugar? What role does sugar play in keeping your body weight normal? What role does sugar play in creating insulin insensitivity? On this subject, they say nothing.

There is one population research study that suggests people who eat higher glycemic foods are at risk for diabetes, but even this link is weak.[20]

People in the medical community need to wake up and begin to publicly acknowledge and take seriously the association between what we put into our mouths and the diseases from which we are likely to die. Diabetes and obesity are out of control and eating sugars and foods that act like sugar contribute to these health problems. Diabetes is the most preventable disease on the planet. No one should suffer through a terrible disease that is almost completely avoidable by what we eat.

Remember that the girl at the pet store in the introduction to this book knew intuitively the best diabetes preventative for my dog: Never let her eat human food. We all need to follow the same advice when it comes to eating sugars and foods that act like sugar.

Heart Disease

We all have a fifty percent chance of dying from heart disease (slightly less if you're a woman). Learning how to prevent this disease should not only be the focus of the medical community, but it should be your focus as well. Once again, if we accept the fact that sugar consumption increases body fat, then we have to at least accept that sugar contributes to heart disease. Excess weight gain is an indirect cause of heart disease. Let's see if we can find any closer links between sugar and heart disease.

There is no doubt that there is a link between diabetes and heart disease. The scientific and medical communities have long acknowledged that people who can't control their blood sugar have a much greater risk of stroke, atherosclerosis, and heart attacks than non-diabetics.

The big question is this: If high blood sugar in a diabetic contributes to heart disease, what happens when someone who isn't diabetic eats sugar? It appears that non-diabetics get heart disease for the very same reasons diabetics get the disease; eating sugars and foods that act like sugar. Sugar consumption certainly leads to an increased risk for the disease[21,22] and eating foods that are low on the glycemic index can certainly reduce the risk of heart disease.[23]

Atherosclerosis (clogging on the arteries) is the result of two primary problems: damage to blood vessels and the repairing of that damage. It all begins when the blood vessels of the heart are damaged. Once the blood vessel is damaged, the body will try to patch the damage. The body uses cholesterol as a sort of band-aid and plugs the damaged blood vessel wall with a cholesterol patch. As you may know, this small cholesterol patch can grow and grow until the whole blood vessel is blocked. When blood flow thorough the vessel stops, the tissue being fed by that blood vessel dies. We know this as a heart attack when it occurs in the heart, but blocked blood vessels can occur anywhere in the body.

Here is another million dollar question: How do blood vessels become damaged in the first place? If you think back to the discussion on protein glycation, you will remember that sugar has the tendency to bind to proteins and blood vessels walls are full of proteins. When sugar binds to proteins on blood vessel walls, this causes damage and may be the first step in the development of heart disease.[24] Doctors can now measure the amount of protein glycation in your body, and new studies suggest that the amount of whole-body protein glycation you have can be used to determine if you have a high or low risk of developing heart disease.[25] You can bypass this test altogether and simply reduce the amount of protein glycation occurring in your body by avoiding sugars and foods that act like sugar in your body.

To be sure, the story of how blood vessels are injured and how that injury leads to heart disease is hotly debated. Sugar damage is only one theory, but as we look at other theories, we would find that sugar can affect all those other possible causes. Let's take a look.

High cholesterol has long been blamed for causing atherosclerosis and even though many people are on cholesterol-lowering drugs, cholesterol is really not the problem. Yes, if you have a very high amount of cholesterol in your body, you are more likely to have clogged arteries, but blaming cholesterol for atherosclerosis is a little like blaming the band-aid for the cut. Either way, if you are concerned about high cholesterol, you can lower your cholesterol by eating lower glycemic meals.[26]

Other theories on why blood vessels become damaged focus on the damage that inflammation or oxidation can cause blood vessels. What is interesting about these theories is that it has been shown that increased amounts of sugar in the blood stream can lead to an increase in oxidation.[27] And, eating foods that have a low glycemic index can not only reduce inflammation,[28] but can also improve endothelial function.[29] As mentioned earlier, researchers can measure endothelial function to determine the elasticity of the blood vessels. Poor endothelial function (low elasticity) is a risk factor for heart disease. While none of these studies are conclusive, it appears that sugar and foods that act like sugar have the potential to impact atherosclerosis.

Of course, heart disease is not all about clogged arteries. High blood pressure is the other major heart-related disease. Once again, people with diabetes and metabolic syndrome are much more likely to have high blood pressure.[30] In fact, having high blood pressure is one of the indicators doctors use to determine if you have metabolic syndrome. Remember that sugar can do damage to the small blood vessels of the body and when this happens in the kidneys, the result is hypertension.[31]

At every step, sugar and foods that act like sugar have the potential to play a role in heart disease. Further studies will, no doubt, help us understand the exact role sugar plays in heart disease and if it is a major cause of heart disease or merely a contributing factor. Imagine the impact on our health if we could reduce this major killer by simply changing the way we eat.

Imagine

Much has been written about the diseases that sugar can cause. It has been suggested that sugar can cause cancer, depression, multiple sclerosis, asthma, arthritis, and various other diseases. While it is tempting to blame sugar for all our ills, many of these claims of sugar's harm have little to no research to support them. The most interesting of the studies focus on the relationship of sugar and cancer, but even these studies are not enough to make any association between sugar foods and the incredible rise in the amount of cancer.

What we do know, without question, is that sugar wreaks havoc on the bodies of people with diabetes. The question of how sugar affects the rest of the people in the world remains. What is obvious from the research presented in this book is that a large amount of sugar consumption is harmful because it represents a dramatic departure from what we, as humans, should be eating.

Imagine, for a moment, a world where diabetes, obesity, and heart disease are uncommon. A world where we all move into old age without having to take a hand full of pills everyday just to survive. Image a world where you wake up every morning full of energy to take on the day.

Even though I have pointed out that medical associations, such as the American Diabetes Association, American Heart Association, and American Cancer Society are hopelessly lost when the subject of sugar arises, I agree with them when they say that up to seventy percent of heart disease, obesity and diabetes can be prevented through proper nutrition and exercise. Think about that!

What you need to know is this: Your health is not in the hands of someone else. You make hundreds of small decisions every day about what to eat and how to live your life. These decisions are important and play themselves out in your health, or lack of it.

Diabetes, obesity, and heart disease are the three diseases I refer to as the sugar triad. Having one of these diseases increase the odds that you will have another one of them. They are all related. They can also all be avoided. By limiting sugars and foods that act like sugar from your diet, you can greatly reduce your risk of ever having any of these diseases. Keeping your blood sugar low is the key, how to accomplish this will be the focus of the last chapter in this book.

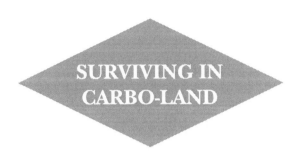

SURVIVING IN CARBO-LAND

Reading this book has been a journey. We have traveled together to some rather strange places. First, we visited a town where little kids are given cigarettes to keep them calm. You then traveled back to 1800 to visit a general store. You visited a field some 10,000 years ago to see what kind of foods might match what your body needs. You found yourself in a high school science class and have journeyed inside your body's cells where you learned how your body adapts to high blood sugar and how sugar alters the way your entire body functions. You have seen the damage that sugar can cause, especially to your blood vessels.

But the strangest place you will ever journey may be the land that you travel through every day: I call that place Carbo-Land. Carbo-Land is the world where grains and sugars have moved from occasional food to becoming the mainstay of our diet. Carbohydrates are everywhere, from billboards, movies and commercials, to your friends, and your mother all tempting you to come and taste the sweetness. Trying to stop eating and drinking sugar foods in Carbo-Land is a little like being an alcoholic working in a bar or a heroin addict working in an opium den. The minute you stop eating sugar and foods that act like sugar, you begin to notice how much our society is geared towards trying to get you to put some sort of carbohydrate into your mouth.

You may have been confused by our time machine's 10,000-year trip into the past, but imagine the opposite. Imagine some cave woman making the trip forward from her time to ours and how very confused she would be. She would undoubtedly be confused by how we choose to live, how we travel, and the many gadgets that surround us. But quite possibly, what may puzzle her most of all would be what we call food.

While most of us assume that the foods we turn to for a meal are the foods human beings have always eaten, the truth is that your dinner plate is dramatically different from what our ancient ancestors ate. One researcher has commented on how much our food choices have changed over time:

> There is surprisingly little overlap between current foods and those of the Paleolithic. We get most of our calories from grains, domesticated livestock, dairy and refined sugars, but pre-agricultural humans ate naturally occurring plant foods and wild game. They used almost no cereal grains and had no dairy foods, no separated oils, no commercial processing, and no sources of "empty calories." People in the Stone Age consumed more animal protein than do current Westerners.[1]

Changing the foods we eat from low-glycemic vegetables and meats to a carbohydrate-laden diet has had dramatic consequences on our health. This is no small point: What we decide to eat determines, to a large extent, how healthy we are and how long we will live. The choices you make every day are reflected in whom you become and what diseases you are likely to have later in life.

You can easily recognize people who have smoked for a long time because their faces and bodies show the destruction caused by cigarettes. That destruction is the result of thousands of little choices made throughout a lifetime. Do you think that a smoker is surprised when a doctor tells them that they have lung cancer? Probably not. Most smokers realize that they are responsible for what happened to their health. People who choose to eat large amounts of sugar foods are just as responsible for their health.

Imagine for a moment that you have a brand new car, but you don't take care of it very well. You may take your car to the car wash occasionally and even vacuum it every once and a while, but you don't change the oil and don't choose the right fuel for the engine. The car is able to run on the fuel you put in it, but it is not what the car needs to function at its best. When the car is new, none of this matters much. As the car gets older, though, it may look just fine from the outside, but the engine is being slowly destroyed by the way you are treating it.

Your body is exactly the same way. You can eat sugars and grains, but they are not the best fuel for your body. As your blood sugar rises every day, it acts the same way that smoke does upon entering a smoker's lungs: it causes damage. The destruction caused by high blood sugar is slow so you don't really notice it... at least not at first. Just because you can't see the damage caused by sugar when you are twenty, thirty, or forty years old, doesn't mean it isn't happening.

You may have heard of the tipping point concept, a point where everything can change at once: Think about a football game where one team is winning and something happens and suddenly the other team begins to win. Your car or your body is exactly like this; they can go for years without showing any damage until one day when everything suddenly falls apart.

Your body can take a large amount of abuse, almost indefinitely, until one day when everything tips the other way and you end up in your doctor's office asking her to fix you.

As I write this, I just got news of a friend of my brother who died of a massive heart attack at the age of 48. He was healthy, cycled to work every day, lived in a small town with very little stress, but he still had a heart attack. Eating sugar and foods that act like sugar is like throwing high-octane fuel into *pipes* that are meant for low-octane fuel. Sugar is too pure, too strong, and it wreaks havoc whenever we decide to eat it. Learning how to eliminate sugar or the harmful effects of sugar can turn the tables on this destruction. Controlling sugar will help you to live the life you always wanted to live: a life full of energy, free from many of the diseases that plague our modern world.

This was never meant to be a diet book with meal plans and recipes; rather, a book to educate you on the addictive qualities and harm that sugar can cause. Other authors do a great job with specific dietary suggestions and you can continue your education by checking the Resource page at the end of the book for further reading. My website, www.olsonnd.com will also have suggestions and advice on how to navigate Carbo-land more effectively. I do, however, want to leave you with three overviews to help you begin your journey. Choose the one that matches your interests, your current health, and your level of commitment.

Plan One

The first plan is the easiest. You have read through the entire book and you understand that sugar and foods that act like sugar have the potential to do harm to your body. You understand this, but you decide to go on doing just what you have been doing and make no changes to your life. You love carbohydrates too much to give them up so you just decide to enjoy your life while you can, knowing full well the dangers involved.

This plan would be akin to a smoker knowing that smoking causes lung cancer and yet continues to smoke. I'm hoping that you don't choose this plan.

Plan Two

The second plan is also easy: remove all sugars and foods that act like sugar from your diet. Well, this plan is easy to say, but not so easy to do. If you really want to break the hold that sugar foods have on you, you have to completely remove all sugars, grains, and starchy vegetables from your diet. You would, therefore, only be eating foods that are low on the glycemic index or, better yet: foods that are below the glycemic index. This is the only real way to break your carbohydrate addiction.

You should seriously consider this plan if you currently have health problems, such as diabetes, heart disease, cancer, or other diseases. You will be surprised how powerful changing the way that you eat can affect your health. You may also want to try this plan if you have a strong family history of heart disease or diabetes.

If you are overweight, you may also want to follow this plan. You can consider removing all sugar foods as the *induction* phase of a weight loss program and you can follow it strictly until you reach your desired weight. Once at your ideal weight, you can switch to the next plan where you learn to keep your blood sugar low while still eating some sugar foods. Be careful though; you can expect to come face to face with your addiction the moment that you put any carbohydrates back into your mouth. Remember, binging is very common when you return to an addiction.

Finally, you may want to try this plan if you are curious. Perhaps you've read through this book, but have not really believed that you are addicted to sugar foods. By trying this plan, you will know in a very short period if you are addicted to sugars and foods that act like sugar. I recommend that everyone try this plan first just to see how well their body responds to good foods and to see just how addicted they are to grains and sugars.

What to Expect

If you decide to remove all sugar foods from your diet, you should be prepared to feel very differently than the way you now feel. At first you will feel worse and then, if you are typical, you will feel better than you have in years.

When you first stop eating and drinking sugar and foods that act like sugar, you are in for a wild ride. Remember that you are a sugar-junkie and you are going to go through withdrawal. For some people, this withdrawal will be mild; for others, they are going to have headaches, flu-like symptoms, mood changes, and other symptoms. And, of course, you are going to have cravings. When you stop eating sugar foods, your body is going to rebel and tell you that you still need them, even if you have just eaten a full meal. If you know these symptoms are going to happen, you can plan and prepare for them. I devote a whole section to cravings and what to do about them later in this chapter.

A common complaint of people who have removed sugar foods from their diet is that they feel dry. What they are experiencing is the loss of water in their body. When you stop putting alien foods into your body, it responds by releasing a lot of the water it has been holding onto. Most people are walking around bloated because they carry a lot of extra water weight. The reason for this is simple. Your body functions by a rule: When you are eating foods that the body identifies as toxic, it will hold onto water to dilute that toxin. I know of a woman who lost thirty pounds in two weeks because she was eating soy (that she was allergic to). The minute she stopped eating soy, she lost all that water weight. Many people who avoid sugars and foods that act like sugar experience some water weight loss.

You may also go through what can only be called a healing reaction. Your body is suddenly working much better than it has in years and your body may take this opportunity to get rid of a lot of junk. You may experience all sorts of illnesses. A cold or flu is common, as are skin disturbances, such as a rash. While you may think this is strange, it is part of the healing process and you shouldn't be alarmed or even rush to treat it. Give it time and the healing reaction will run its course. You will come out on the other side feeling better than you have in a long time.

While removing sugar foods may be difficult at first – and you may experience some discomfort – you also want to be prepared to feel much better than you do right now. Many people who begin this kind of diet plan say that they feel awful at first, but then soon feel surprisingly better. Choosing to forgo all grains, sugars, and other high-glycemic foods is going to put you on the path towards a longer and healthier life. Those who make the shift to a better way of eating report sleeping better, having increased energy, and often lose weight.

High Protein?

Throughout this book you have heard me say that you should avoid sugars and foods that act like sugar. The immediate thought in most people's minds when they read "remove all carbohydrates" is that I'm suggesting a high protein diet. I'm not. While I don't think that eating a large amount of protein is as harmful as some health professional would have you believe, I would suggest two things to think about when you choose to remove sugar foods from your diet.

The first is protein quality. There is a great difference between bacon and wild-caught salmon, or a fast-food hamburger and a grass-fed buffalo. Choose your proteins wisely. If you eat proteins from organically grown sources, rather than from grain-fed animals, you will be getting a very different protein than someone who is stopping by fast-food restaurants for a hamburger. Meat from grain-fed animals has a higher fat content than non-grain-fed meat. Organic foods have also consistently been shown to have higher amounts of essential nutrients compared to conventionally grown foods which have had their goodness destroyed by antibiotics, growth hormones, additives, and preservatives.

The other thing you should know is that I'm not recommending that you increase your protein intake. I generally suggest that people keep their protein intake about the same. So the question becomes, what do you fill your plate with? I suggest that you replace all of your grains and sugars with vegetables and fruits. If you would normally reach for some bread at dinner, try having green beans, broccoli, or another vegetable. Instead of reaching for potato chips to snack on, try an apple or other low glycemic fruit (see: Flipping the Pyramid, later in this book). Every place where you would normally have a high octane sugar food, choose something whole and fresh.

SCOTT OLSON

Replacing carbohydrates with vegetables and fruits is one of the healthiest things you can do for yourself.

Plan Overview

Avoid:

- All grains
- All sugars
- High glycemic vegetables (starches)
- High glycemic fruits

Eat:

- Low glycemic vegetables
- Low glycemic fruits
- Proteins: meats, nuts, beans

Plan Three

Most people will fall somewhere between plan one and plan two: They want to try to do something different and reduce the impact sugar has on their lives, but they are not willing to give up all grains and sugars.

While there is no doubt that avoiding all sugars, grains, and starchy vegetables is by far the best way to health, you can still create a plan designed to keep your blood sugar low without cutting out all carbohydrates. The only downside of this plan is that you are going to constantly be battling with your sugar addiction because you are still eating foods that act like sugar. This is a little like trying to smoke only one cigarette a day or having only one beer a day for alcoholics. Can it be done? Yes,

145

it can, but you have to be very careful that you don't return to your old ways of eating.

Eat with the Glycemic Index in Mind

In order to make plan three effective, you need to keep your blood sugar low. To keep your blood sugar low, we have to go back to the glycemic index to develop an eating strategy. So far, we have been talking about how single foods affect blood sugar levels; this is the best use of the glycemic index. Unfortunately, the glycemic index is not that helpful in predicting what happens when you take a low glycemic food and mix it with a high glycemic index food, as you would in any meal. Sometimes mixing a high-glycemic food with a low-glycemic food increases your blood sugar dramatically while at other times it doesn't. So what good is the glycemic index if it can't predict the way all foods will react when we eat them?

The glycemic index provides general information about how to keep blood sugar levels low, but it does not guarantee what happens when you combine foods. However, after looking at thousands of foods and how they affect blood sugar, we can determine certain general principles about the characteristics of foods that can help to keep blood sugar low.

General Glycemic Index Principles

Here are the general glycemic index principles:

- Sugars, grains, and starches increase blood sugar

This we already know. Since sugars, grains, and starches increase blood sugar, we have to learn what can keep your blood sugar low. Here is what the glycemic index has taught us that will help keep blood our sugar low:

- Fat
- Fiber
- Protein

These three types of foods will keep sugars from being absorbed quickly and keep your blood sugar low. What you are doing with this plan is surrounding any sugar food with other foods that can keep your blood sugar from dramatically increasing. Plan 3 way of eating looks like this:

- **Never eat sugar or foods that act like sugar without a fat, fiber, or protein somewhere in the meal.** So, that afternoon soda, bag of chips, or candy bar, I would still say to keep out of your diet because eating them alone will raise your blood sugar too high. If you simply cannot do without these sugary foods, eat them during or right after a meal that contains fat, protein, and fiber. For example, if you want to have some bread, choose whole grain bread (for the fiber) and make a peanut butter or meat sandwich (for the fat and protein). The more vegetables you can eat with the bread, such as a salad or lettuce on the sandwich (increasing the fiber), the better. Or, put another way: **Never put a high glycemic sugar food in your mouth unless it is near some sort of fat, fiber, or protein.**

Here are some other suggestions to make this plan work for you:

- **Stop the Soda:** I've mentioned this in many parts of this book, but just to make sure that you have heard me, I'm saying it again. **Don't ever pick up a soda again; avoid it like poison.**

- **Stop the Sugar**: While you can probably keep your blood sugar level low even if you eat foods that act like sugar by incorporating a fat, fiber, or protein, it's important to stay away from the real, concentrated table sugar as much as possible. Even though I suggest you should stay away from sugar completely, you may be tempted from time to time to have something sweet (like having cake on your birthday). The best way to do this is to eat the sugary snack immediately after your meal, rather than several hours later. Your blood sugar will still rise, but by having your sweet treat right after your meal, you will be helping to keep your blood sugar lower than if you ate the cake hours later.

- **Eat grains as whole as possible:** If you are going to eat grains, it's vital to eat grains in whole form as much as possible. This means eating grains as most people eat rice – simply boil the grain and eat it with your meal. Every grain can be prepared this way, but look for different grains such as barley, quinoa, teff, amaranth, and others. If you can't boil and eat all your grains, then choose the next best thing. Whole wheat bread, for example, is better than white bread and oatmeal is better than bread made with oat flour. Luckily, pasta – an easy to prepare grain –tends to be low on the glycemic index.

- **Replace Sugar Foods with Vegetables or Fruits:** If you are thinking about having some bread, rice, pasta, or any other carbohydrate with your meal, consider replacing it with a low-glycemic index vegetable or fruit. I call this kind of eating "flipping the pyramid," a term coined by my nine-year-old who pointed out that the food pyramid she'd been given at school was upside-down and needed to be flipped because it recommends more grains, meat, and vegetables at the bottom.

To understand what I mean by flipping the pyramid, take a look at a typical food pyramid:

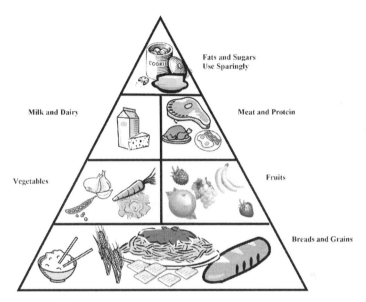

Part of this pyramid is correct; you should use sugars sparingly, if at all. But a food pyramid that takes into account what human beings *should* be eating would look more like this:

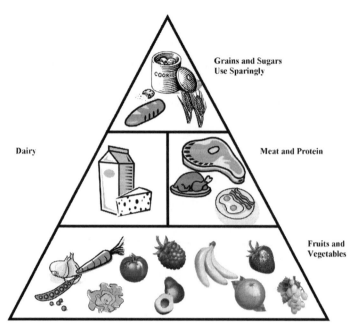

Most of your diet should be comprised of fruits and vegetables, with meat and proteins making up the remainder. Grain and sugars can be part of your diet if they are consumed sparingly and occasionally.

And, finally, the last suggestion to make this plan work:

- **Eat More Often**: While this might be counter to what you believe, research illustrates that blood sugar levels stay steady when you eat many meals throughout the day, rather than two or three large meals.

Plan Overview

Avoid:

- Sugar, high glycemic vegetables (starches) and high glycemic fruits when eaten alone

Eat:

- A vegetarian-type diet (high in fruits and vegetables) supplemented by healthy proteins
- Low glycemic vegetables
- Low glycemic fruits
- More fiber-rich foods
- Proteins: beans, meats, and nuts

The key to plan three: Avoid sugar foods when you can, but if you eat them, make sure that you eat them with a protein, fiber, or fat in the same meal. If weight loss is your goal, I would suggest that you go with the second plan first and once you are at your desired weight, you can switch to plan three.

What to Do about Cravings

Whether you choose plan two or plan three, you will probably experience cravings. Sugar cravings are your brain's way of tricking you; they make you think that you need something you don't. Your mind is used to being *turned on* by the sugars in the foods that you have been eating and it wants the same stimulation over and over again. You are a sugar junkie and your mind is trying to convince you that you are going to die if you don't put a doughnut in your mouth. Don't believe it!

If there is anything that will derail your forward progress, it is your old addiction coming back to haunt you. While many professionals who talk about addictions will tell you that your addictions go away after three to seven days, I have never believed this advice. I think once addicted, always addicted; most addicts would tell you the same. So instead of chastising yourself for your addiction and for how weak you feel when you crave something sweet, prepare yourself for a battle that will last a lifetime.

The first thing you should do is to remove from your house, car, and work place anything that will tempt you. Everyone has their weaknesses and you know yours. Grab whatever you are most tempted by and remove it from your reach. If you still choose to eat foods that act like sugar, you will be tempting yourself every day; this is sort of like smoking one cigarette every day. Some people can do it, but most find this very difficult. Whenever you have a bad day, you will have easy access to your addiction. While keeping your addiction around makes it difficult to keep from binging, you can still do it.

Try to think ahead about what you are going to do and how you are going to handle the bad day, the celebration, or your monthly cycle (for women), when the desire to binge will often rear its ugly head. Preparing yourself in advance can help you take charge of the situation.

Here are some practical tips:

- **Eat often**: This not only helps balance your blood sugar level, but it also lessens the number of cravings you will have. While you may feel silly eating lunch at ten o'clock in the morning and having another lunch around noon, and yet another meal at two o'clock, having three small lunches is a great way to balance your blood sugar level.
- **Eat dried fruit:** Many people crave sweet foods after they eat. Eating something like fruit or a dried

fruit following a meal can help. Don't overdo it, though.

- **Salad greens:** Many grocery stores stock mixed salad greens. Eating these before a meal tends to fill people up; they are also loaded with vitamins and other nutrients so it's a great two-for-one filler-upper!
- **Exercise:** If you feel that craving-monster beginning to creep up on you, go for a walk. Exercise not only gets you out of the kitchen and onto the street and away from your temptations, it has also been shown to reduce cravings.
- **Brush your teeth:** Brushing gives you a sweet taste and many people don't feel like eating once their mouths have been cleaned.
- **Drink water:** Sometimes cravings get mixed up in your brain and what your body really needs is water and not sugar. Try drinking a glass of water when your cravings begin.
- **Try supplementing:** Supplements can help with cravings, including:
  - o **Amino acids:** Tyrosine, phenylalanine, gamma-aminobutyric acid (GABA), tryptophan, and glutamine can help. Glutamine is sweet-tasting and can be placed under the tongue after a meal or between meals to calm cravings.
  - o **B-complex**: A good mixture of B-vitamins is essential for reducing cravings.
  - o **Minerals**: Some researchers claim that cravings are based on the need for minerals in our bodies. This is especially true of chromium, which has also been shown to help balance blood sugar levels.
  - o **Gymnema**: This herb has been shown to help with blood sugar control and cravings.

- o **A good multi-vitamin**: Multi-vitamins can help quell cravings. Many include the B-vitamins and minerals (as mentioned above).
- **Remember, it is just a craving:** You don't have to be a slave to your cravings. You have probably eaten recently so you are not going to starve – even though your brain is trying to convince you that you are. Often, you can out-wait your craving and it will go away.

The main thing to remember is that if you fall off the plan and cravings get the best of you, keep bringing yourself back, over and over again. Consider your fall from the wagon to be like a drinking binge, from which you return to healthy living habits as soon as you can.

The End of the Journey

Okay, you can unbuckle your seat belts and step off the ride. I hope that you have enjoyed your trip. Living in Carbo-Land can be very difficult. Remember, learning how to keep your blood sugar level low is one of the keys to a long and healthy life.

One of the reasons cigarette smoking, or any other addiction, is so tempting is that you cannot see the results of the destruction these addictions cause for a long time. If you took one puff of a cigarette and discovered immediately that it was difficult to breathe, and your skin began to wrinkle, and your heart was damaged, you would likely never take another puff again. But somehow, when the damage takes its sweet time to make an appearance, people are willing to trade their lives for a short pick-me-up and a good feeling.

As recently as one hundred years ago, most people died of infectious diseases. Through improvements in sanitation, better nutrition, and miracle drugs, we now lead much longer lives. But as infectious diseases have reduced in numbers, we are now faced with an epidemic of chronic diseases, such as cancer, heart disease, and diabetes. What you need to do in order to combat long term diseases is realize, just as a smoker must do, that your health comes down to choices. A smoker makes the decision to pull a cigarette out of the pack, bring it to her lips, light it, and inhale, hundreds of thousands of times. One cigarette does not hurt you; it is the thousands of cigarettes over a long period of time that causes the damage. Sugar is no different. It tastes good, you feel good when eating it, and it makes you momentarily happy. All the while, sugar foods are slowly destroying your body.

Throughout the book I have mentioned that human beings are better suited to the foods our cavemen ancestors ate. You may think that I would suggest that we go back to this time, but nothing could be further from the truth. While the food choices available to our ancestors were a perfect match for our bodies, their lives were tough, brutal and short.

In the world we live in today, we are in a position to feed ourselves better than any human beings have ever been fed but, somehow, we don't. We have, as a culture, decided to prioritize cheap tasty food that is easy for farmers to farm, manufacturers to manufacture, and stores to store, instead of prioritizing food that is best suited for human growth and thriving. This needs to change.

Who you are when you grow older is the result of all the decisions that you have made throughout your lifetime. Medical professionals all agree that many diseases (perhaps as many as seventy percent) are the result of lifestyle choices and that you can avoid these diseases by the choices you make. Read that again: your health is in your hands. You are the one who decides if you get diabetes, heart disease, or cancer. Take the time to make the right decisions for you and your miraculous body.

I wish you the best on your personal journey.

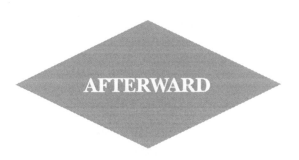

AFTERWARD

You may have noticed that there is an ND after my name and not an MD. The ND stands for Naturopathic Doctor. I'm often asked what kind of doctor a Naturopath is, so here is an explanation:

Naturopaths: The Doctors of the Future

After being shuttled in and out of a doctor's appointment in less than 10 minutes, you might have wished for something better. You may have also wished that your doctor could not only prescribe the drugs you need, but also talk to you about what you can do to heal yourself using diet, nutrition, herbs, vitamins, and homeopathy, or other natural healing methods.

Maybe, you think, the doctor of the future will have a more balanced approach and be your partner in health.

The doctor of the future is already here. Naturopathic Doctors (NDs), who have attended licensed naturopathic colleges, have an understanding of both standard medical practice and natural healing methods. NDs are doctors who are trained very similarly to medical doctors, but who have an entirely different approach to health and healing that recognizes the self-healing potential inside all of us. Naturopaths have the ability to help you decide between either medical or natural healing choices, depending on your situation. Naturopaths work to un-cover the root cause of the disease and not simply mask the problem by making symptoms go away with drug therapy.

Naturopaths recognize that there are many routes to health in-cluding exercise, diet, digestion, and elimination and they use natural healing methods such as herbs, vitamins, homeopathy, nutrition and much more. In short, naturopathic doctors treat the whole person. Naturopathic doctors take the time to edu-cate the patient both on their disease and on ways to become healthier. They recognize that preventing diseases is often much easier than treating them.

While there currently aren't many naturopaths, their numbers are growing. The licensing of Naturopaths is different in each state so they may not be able to prescribe drugs or perform cer-tain procedures depending on which state you are in. Check the Resource page at the end of the book, or my website www.olsonnd.com for help finding a naturopathic doctor in your area.

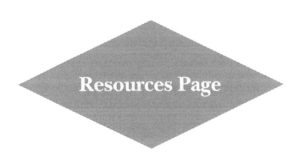

Resources Page

I am hoping that this book is just the beginning of your journey towards a more health life. You have more control over your health than you may realize. The choices you make every day have a powerful effect on how healthy you are later in your life.

One of the best ways to keep making good choices is to make a study of health. I encourage you to read more books, visit websites, and find a health practitioner that can help guide you through the maze of health medicine.

The following resources are a great place to start:

Web

- You can find me on the web at: www.olsonnd.com, where you can comment on blog topics, ask me questions and stay informed on the latest sugar topics.
- I have a page on Facebook, where you can join in the conversation, ask questions, and get support for dealing with sugar addiction.

Other great websites:

- Find a Naturopath in your area at the American Association of Naturopathic Physicians: www.naturopathic.org
- For more on Weston Price and the changes that occur when we switch from traditional diets: www.westona-price.org
- Joseph Mercola is a medical doctor who is a leader in health education. His website, www.mercola.com is a wealth of information on health and healing.

Books

Books on Sugar:

- *Sugar Blues* by William Dufty: This is the classic book on the problems with sugar. Written in 1975, it is still pertinent today.

Food Choices

- *The No-Grain Diet* by Joseph Mercola: A great book to help you to learn to live without grains, it has a lot of dietary suggestions.
- *Traditional Foods Are Your Best Medicine: Improving Health and Longevity with Native Nutrition* by Ronald F. Schmid: This book changed my life, it was the first book I read where I read about Paleolithic diets.
- *The Paleolithic Prescription: A Program of Diet and Exercise and a Design for Living* by Boyd, Eaton, Shostak, and Konner: Another great book.
- *The Omnivore's Dilemma: A Natural History of Four Meals* by Michael Pollan: Michael Pollan's exhaustively re-

searched and wonderful text has a lot to say about all that has changed in our diets.

Artificial Sweeteners

- *Sweet Deception: Why Splenda, NutraSweet, and the FDA May Be Hazardous to Your Health* by Mercola and Pearsall: a great read, full of convincing evidence for avoiding these hazardous non-foods.
- *Aspartame: Is it Safe?* by H.J. Roberts: A classic text on the problems with artificial sweeteners.

Cook Books

- *Nourishing Traditions*, by Sally Fallon: This is more than just a cookbook, and a great read.
- *Carbohydrate Addict's Lifespan Program* by Heller and Heller: This book is also more than a cookbook, but has some great suggestions for reducing sugar food's impact on your blood sugar.

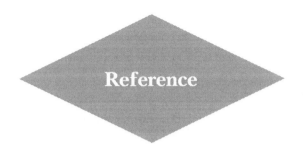

Reference

INTRODUCTION

1 Sugar Association website, accessed 4/20/2008: http://www.sugar.org/media/rss/?id=540

2 Sugar Association website, accessed 4/20/2008: http://www.sugar.org/media/rss/?id=540

3 Eaton SB, Strassman BI, Nesse RM, et al: Evolutionary health promotion. Prev Med. 2002 Feb;34(2):109-18.

4 Eaton SB, Strassman BI, Nesse RM, et al: Evolutionary health promotion. Prev Med. 2002 Feb;34(2):109-18.

THE HISTORY OF YOUR DINNER

1 Eaton SB, Strassman BI, Nesse RM, et al: Evolutionary health promotion. Prev Med. 2002 Feb;34(2):109-18.

LET'S TALK CARBS

1 Bray GA, Nielsen SJ, Popkin BM: Consumption of high-fructose corn syrup in beverages may play a role in the epidemic of obesity. Am J Clin Nutr. 2004 Apr;79(4):537-43.

2 Stanhope KL, Havel PJ: Fructose consumption: potential mechanisms for its effects to increase visceral adiposity and induce dyslipidemia and insulin resistance. Curr Opin Lipidol. 2008 Feb;19(1):16-24.

3 Ouyang X, Cirillo P, Sautin Y, et al: Fructose consumption as a risk factor for non-alcoholic fatty liver disease. J Hepatol. 2008 Jun;48(6):993-9.

4 Harrington S. The role of sugar-sweetened beverage consumption in adolescent obesity: a review of the literature. J Sch Nurs. 2008 Feb;24(1):3-12.

5 Malik VS, Schulze MB, Hu FBL Intake of sugar-sweetened beverages and weight gain: a systematic review. Am J Clin Nutr. 2006 Aug;84(2):274-88.

6 Wolf A, Bray GA, Popkin BM: A short history of beverages and how our body treats them. Obes Rev. 2008 Mar;9(2):151-64.

7 Harrington S. The role of sugar-sweetened beverage consumption in adolescent obesity: a review of the literature. J Sch Nurs. 2008 Feb;24(1):3-12.

SUGAR MAGNET

1 Sugar Association website, accessed 4/20/2008: http://www.sugar.org/media/rss/?id=540

2 Spangler R, Wittkowski KM, Goddard NL, et al: Opiate-like effects of sugar on gene expression in reward areas of the rat brain. Brain Res Mol Brain Res. 2004 May 19;124(2):134-42.

3 Wideman CH, Nadzam GR, Murphy HM: Implications of an animal model of sugar addiction, withdrawal and relapse for human health. Nutr Neurosci. 2005 Oct-Dec;8(5-6):269-76.

4 Erlanson-Albertsson C: Sugar triggers our reward-system. Sweets release opiates which stimulates the appetite for sucrose–insulin can depress it. Lakartidningen. 2005 May 23-29;102(21):1620-2, 1625, 1627.

5 Colantuoni C, Rada P, McCarthy J, et al: Evidence that intermittent, excessive sugar intake causes endogenous opioid dependence. Obes Res. 2002 Jun;10(6):478-88.

6 Galic MA, Persinger MA: Voluminous sucrose consumption in female rats: increased "nippiness" during periods of sucrose removal and possible oestrus periodicity. Psychol Rep. 2002 Feb;90(1):58-60.

7 Gosnell BA. Sucrose intake predicts rate of acquisition of cocaine self-administration. Psychopharmacology (Berl). 2000 Apr;149(3):286-92.

8 Peciña S, Schulkin J, Berridge KC: Nucleus accumbens corticotropin-releasing factor increases cue-triggered motivation for sucrose reward:

paradoxical positive incentive effects in stress? BMC Biol. 2006 Apr 13;4:8.

9   Rada P, Avena NM, Hoebel BG. Daily bingeing on sugar repeatedly releases dopamine in the accumbens shell. Neuroscience. 2005;134(3):737-44.

10 Avena NM, Long KA, Hoebel BG: Sugar-dependent rats show enhanced responding for sugar after abstinence: evidence of a sugar deprivation effect. Physiol Behav. 2005 Mar 16;84(3):359-62.

11 Colantuoni C, Schwenker J, McCarthy J, et al: Excessive sugar intake alters binding to dopamine and mu-opioid receptors in the brain. Neuroreport. 2001 Nov 16;12(16):3549-52.

12 Krahn D, Grossman J, Henk H, et al: Sweet intake, sweet-liking, urges to eat, and weight change: relationship to alcohol dependence and abstinence. Addict Behav. 2006 Apr;31(4):622-31. Epub 2005 Jun 29.

13 Avena NM, Bocarsly ME, Rada P, et al: After daily bingeing on a sucrose solution, food deprivation induces anxiety and accumbens dopamine/acetylcholine imbalance. Physiol Behav. 2008 Jun 9;94(3):309-15.

14 Lenoir M, Serre F, Cantin L, Ahmed SH: Intense sweetness surpasses cocaine reward. PLoS ONE. 2007 Aug 1;2(1):e698.

15 Avena NM.Examining the addictive-like properties of binge eating using an animal model of sugar dependence. Exp Clin Psychopharmacol. 2007 Oct;15(5):481-91.

16 Pelchat ML. Of human bondage: food craving, obsession, compulsion, and addiction. Physiol Behav. 2002 Jul;76(3):347-52.

17 Kampov-Polevoy AB, Garbutt JC, Janowsky DS: Association between preference for sweets and excessive alcohol intake: a review of animal and human studies. Alcohol Alcohol. 1999 May-Jun;34(3):386-95.

18 Avena NM, Rada P, Hoebel BG: Evidence for sugar addiction: behavioral and neurochemical effects of intermittent, excessive sugar intake. Neurosci Biobehav Rev. 2008;32(1):20-39. Epub 2007 May 18.

SUGAR MEETS BODY

1   Bantle JP: Clinical aspects of sucrose and fructose metabolism. Diabetes Care. 1989 Jan;12(1):56-61; discussion 81-2.

2 Narayan KM, Boyle JP, Thompson TJ, et al: Lifetime risk for diabetes mellitus in the United States. JAMA. 2003 Oct 8;290(14):1884-90.

3 Narayan KM, Boyle JP, Thompson TJ, et al: Lifetime risk for diabetes mellitus in the United States. JAMA. 2003 Oct 8;290(14):1884-90.

4 Schneider S, Manolopoulos K, Klein HH: The metabolic syndrome. Versicherungsmedizin. 2007 Sep 1;59(3):115-9.

5 Bessesen DH. The role of carbohydrates in insulin resistance. J Nutr. 2001 Oct;131(10):2782S-2786S.

6 Daly M: Sugars, insulin sensitivity, and the postprandial state. Am J Clin Nutr. 2003 Oct;78(4):865S-872S.

7 Lustig RH. The 'skinny' on childhood obesity: how our western environment starves kids' brains. Pediatr Ann. 2006 Dec;35(12):898-902, 905-7.

8 Miller A, Adeli K: Dietary fructose and the metabolic syndrome. Curr Opin Gastroenterol. 2008 Mar;24(2):204-9.

9 Friedman EA: Advanced glycosylated end products and hyperglycemia in the pathogenesis of diabetic complications. Diabetes Care. 1999 Mar;22 Suppl 2:B65-71.

10 Goldin A, Beckman JA, Schmidt AM, et al: Advanced glycation end products: sparking the development of diabetic vascular injury. Circulation. 2006 Aug 8;114(6):597-605.

11 Kanwar YS, Wada J, Sun L, et al: Diabetic nephropathy: mechanisms of renal disease progression.
Exp Biol Med (Maywood). 2008 Jan;233(1):4-11.

12 Thornalley PJ: Glycation in diabetic neuropathy: characteristics, consequences, causes, and therapeutic options. Int Rev Neurobiol. 2002;50:37-57.

13 Stitt AW, Frizzell N, Thorpe SR: Advanced glycation and advanced lipoxidation: possible role in initiation and progression of diabetic retinopathy. Curr Pharm Des. 2004;10(27):3349-60.

14 Misciagna G, De Michele G, Cisternino AM, et al: Dietary carbohydrates and glycated proteins in the blood in non diabetic subjects. J Am Coll Nutr. 2005 Feb;24(1):22-9.

15 Livesey G, Taylor R, Hulshof T, Howlett J: Glycemic response and health--a systematic review and meta-analysis: relations between dietary glycemic

properties and health outcomes. Am J Clin Nutr. 2008 Jan;87(1):258S-268S.

16 Colaco CA.Sugar and coronary heart disease, a molecular explanation. J R Soc Med. 1993 Apr;86(4):243.

17 Price CL, Knight SC: Advanced glycation: a novel outlook on atherosclerosis. Curr Pharm Des. 2007;13(36):3681-7.

18 Cersosimo E, DeFronzo RA: Insulin resistance and endothelial dysfunction: the road map to cardiovascular diseases. Diabetes Metab Res Rev. 2006 Nov-Dec;22(6):423-36.

19 Ganda OP, Arkin CF: Hyperfibrinogenemia. An important risk factor for vascular complications in diabetes. Diabetes Care. 1992 Oct;15(10):1245-50.

20 Ezzati M, Lopez AD: Regional, disease specific patterns of smoking-attributable mortality in 2000. Tob Control. 2004 Dec;13(4):388-95.

21 Roglic G, Unwin N, Bennett PH, et al: The burden of mortality attributable to diabetes: realistic estimates for the year 2000. Diabetes Care. 2005 Sep;28(9):2130-5.

22 Atlas of Heart Disease and Stroke, WHO, Sept. 2004

23 Johnson RJ, Segal MS, Sautin Y, et al: Potential role of sugar (fructose) in the epidemic of hypertension, obesity and the metabolic syndrome, diabetes, kidney disease, and cardiovascular disease. Am J Clin Nutr. 2007 Oct;86(4):899-906.

24 Guerci B, Böhme P, Kearney-Schwartz A, et al: Endothelial dysfunction and type 2 diabetes. Part 2: altered endothelial function and the effects of treatments in type 2 diabetes mellitus. Diabetes Metab. 2001 Sep;27(4 Pt 1):436-47.

25 Johnson RJ, Segal MS, Sautin Y, et al: Potential role of sugar (fructose) in the epidemic of hypertension, obesity and the metabolic syndrome, diabetes, kidney disease, and cardiovascular disease. Am J Clin Nutr. 2007 Oct;86(4):899-906.

FOODS THAT ACT LIKE SUGAR

1 The Backbone of History: Health and Nutrition in the Western Hemisphere by Richard H. Steckel (Ed.), Jerome C. Rose (Ed.)

ARTIFICIAL SWEETENERS

1 Soffritti M, Belpoggi F, Tibaldi E, et al: Life-span exposure to low doses of aspartame beginning during prenatal life increases cancer effects in rats. Environ Health Perspect. 2007 Sep;115(9):1293-7.

2 Belpoggi F, Soffritti M, Padovani M, et al: Results of long-term carcinogenicity bioassay on Sprague-Dawley rats exposed to aspartame administered in feed. Ann N Y Acad Sci. 2006 Sep;1076:559-77.

3 Food Chemical News, June 12, 1995, Page 27.

4 Patel RM, Sarma R, Grimsley E: Popular sweetener sucralose as a migraine trigger. Headache. 2006 Sep;46(8):1303-4.

5 Lavin JH, French SJ, Read NW: The effect of sucrose- and aspartame-sweetened drinks on energy intake, hunger and food choice of female, moderately restrained eaters. Int J Obes Relat Metab Disord. 1997 Jan;21(1):37-42.

DISEASE CONNECTION

1 American Diabetes Association website, accessed 5/2/2008: http://www.diabetes.org/for-parents-and-kids/diabetes-care/sugar.jsp

2 Nuttall FQ, Gannon MC: Sucrose and disease. Diabetes Care. 1981 Mar-Apr;4(2):305-10.

3 American Dietetic Association website, accessed on 5/2/2008: http://www.eatright.org/cps/rde/xchg/ada/hs.xsl/home_13071_ENU_HTML.htm

4 Report of a Joint FAO/WHO Consultation. Carbohydrates in human nutrition. FAO Food and Nutrition Paper 66. Geneva: World Health Organization; 1998

5 Bloch AS: Low carbohydrate diets, pro: time to rethink our current strategies. Nutr Clin Pract. 2005 Feb;20(1):3-12.

6 Stanhope KL, Havel PJ: Fructose consumption: potential mechanisms for its effects to increase visceral adiposity and induce dyslipidemia and insulin resistance. Curr Opin Lipidol. 2008 Feb;19(1):16-24.

7 Englyst KN, Englyst HN: Carbohydrate bioavailability. Br J Nutr. 2005 Jul;94(1):1-11.

8 Galic MA, Persinger MA: Voluminous sucrose consumption in female rats: increased "nippiness" during periods of sucrose removal and possible oestrus periodicity. Psychol Rep. 2002 Feb;90(1):58-60.

9 Warren JM, Henry CJ, Simonite V: Low glycemic index breakfasts and reduced food intake in preadolescent children. Pediatrics. 2003 Nov;112(5):e414.

10 Galgani J, Aguirre C, Díaz E: Acute effect of meal glycemic index and glycemic load on blood glucose and insulin responses in humans. Nutr J. 2006 Sep 5;5:22.

11 Livesey G, Taylor R, Hulshof T, Howlett J: Glycemic response and health--a systematic review and meta-analysis: relations between dietary glycemic properties and health outcomes. Am J Clin Nutr. 2008 Jan;87(1):258S-268S.

12 Livesey G: Low-glycaemic diets and health: implications for obesity. Proc Nutr Soc. 2005 Feb;64(1):105-13.

13 Thomas DE, Elliott EJ, Baur L.: Low glycaemic index or low glycaemic load diets for overweight and obesity. Cochrane Database Syst Rev. 2007 Jul 18;(3):CD005105.

14 Misra A, Ganda OP: Migration and its impact on adiposity and type 2 diabetes. Nutrition. 2007 Sep;23(9):696-708.

15 Henriksen HB, Kolset SO: Sugar intake and public health. Tidsskr Nor Laegeforen. 2007 Sep 6;127(17):2259-62.

16 National Diabetes Information Clearing House, accessed 5/9/2008: http://diabetes.niddk.nih.gov/dm/pubs/statistics/index.htm

17 Narayan KM, Boyle JP, Thompson TJ, et al: Lifetime risk for diabetes mellitus in the United States. JAMA. 2003 Oct 8;290(14):1884-90.

18 Howlett J, Ashwell M: Glycemic response and health: summary of a workshop. Am J Clin Nutr. 2008 Jan;87(1):212S-216S.

19 Steyn NP, Mann J, Bennett PH, et al: Diet, nutrition and the prevention of type 2 diabetes. Public Health Nutr. 2004 Feb;7(1A):147-65.

20 Sartorelli DS, Cardoso MA: Association between dietary carbohydrates and type 2 diabetes mellitus: epidemiological evidence, Arq Bras Endocrinol Metabol. 2006 Jun;50(3):415-26.

21 Barclay AW, Petocz P, McMillan-Price J, et al: Glycemic index, glycemic load, and chronic disease risk–a meta-analysis of observational studies. Am J Clin Nutr. 2008 Mar;87(3):627-37.

22 Dickinson S, Brand-Miller J: Glycemic index, postprandial glycemia and cardiovascular disease.Curr Opin Lipidol. 2005 Feb;16(1):69-75.

23 Brand-Miller J, Dickinson S, Barclay A, et al: The glycemic index and cardiovascular disease risk. Curr Atheroscler Rep. 2007 Dec;9(6):479-85.

24 Colaco CA.Sugar and coronary heart disease, a molecular explanation. J R Soc Med. 1993 Apr;86(4):243.

25 Misciagna G, De Michele G, Trevisan M: Non enzymatic glycated proteins in the blood and cardiovascular disease. Curr Pharm Des. 2007;13(36):3688-95.

26 Leeds AR: Glycemic index and heart disease. Am J Clin Nutr. 2002 Jul;76(1):286S-9S.

27 Pennathur S, Heinecke JW: Mechanisms for oxidative stress in diabetic cardiovascular disease. Antioxid Redox Signal. 2007 Jul;9(7):955-69.

28 Schulze MB, Hoffmann K, Manson JE, et al: Dietary pattern, inflammation, and incidence of type 2 diabetes in women. Am J Clin Nutr. 2005 Sep;82(3):675-84; quiz 714-5.

29 Guerci B, Böhme P, Kearney-Schwartz A, et al: Endothelial dysfunction and type 2 diabetes. Part 2: altered endothelial function and the effects of treatments in type 2 diabetes mellitus. Diabetes Metab. 2001 Sep;27(4 Pt 1):436-47.

30 Bakris GL: Current perspectives on hypertension and metabolic syndrome. J Manag Care Pharm. 2007 Jun;13(5 Suppl):S3-5.

SURVIVING IN CARBO-LAND

31 Thomas MC, Forbes JM, Cooper ME. Advanced glycation end products and diabetic nephropathy. Am J Ther. 2005 Nov-Dec;12(6):562-72.

1 Eaton SB, Strassman BI, Nesse RM, et al: Evolutionary health promotion. Prev Med. 2002 Feb;34(2):109-18.

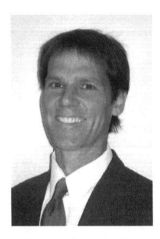

About the Author

Dr. Scott is a naturopathic doctor and a specialist in diet, nutrition, and alternative medicine. He is the author of numerous articles on health, medicine, and alternative medicine. He is available as an expert in health and alternative medicine for interviews and conferences.

Dr. Scott holds a bachelor of arts from Adams State College in Colorado and a doctorate from the National College of Naturopathic medicine in Portland, Oregon; he resides in Colorado with his wife and three children.

If you want to contact Dr. Scott with a questions or a suggestion for improving this text, please contact him at:

support@olsonnd.com

Visit his website at: www.olsonnd.com

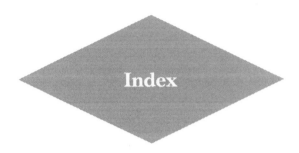

Index

B

C

F

Fatty liver, 50

Feed-forward cycle, 63–64

Fiber, 126, 147

Food and Drug Administration (FDA), 13, 109, 112, 113

Food pyramid, 149

Free radicals, 87, 91

Fructose, 39, 41, 49–51, 90, 123

G

Gateway drug, sugar as, 69

Genetics, and human diet, 21–22, 26–27, 32–33, 101–102, 114, 138

Ghrelin, 83

Glucometer, 50

Glucose, 38, 39, 41, 49–51, 100

Glycated proteins, 87, 88–90, 125, 132

Glycemia, see Blood sugar

Glycemic Index, 44, 98–101, 103–106

diets and, 146–150

diseases and, 123–127

principles of, 146–148

Grains, see Carbohydrates

H

Heart disease, 7, 90–91, 92, 93–95, 131–133

High blood pressure, see Hypertension

High cholesterol, 132–133

High fructose corn syrup (HFCS), 48–51, 90

History

of artificial sweeteners, 108–109

of cigarettes, 1, 4–5, 7, 10–12

of dinner, 25–27

of human diet, 27–34

of sugar, 45–48

Honey, 45

S

2462697

Made in the USA